100 Questions & Answers About Multiple Sclerosis
Second Edition

William A. Sheremata, MD, FRCPC, FACP
Professor of Neurology
Miller School of Medicine
University of Miami
Miami, FL

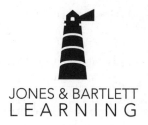

JONES & BARTLETT
LEARNING

World Headquarters

Jones & Bartlett Learning
40 Tall Pine Drive
Sudbury, MA 01776
978-443-5000
info@jblearning.com
www.jblearning.com

Jones & Bartlett Learning
Canada
6339 Ormindale Way
Mississauga, Ontario L5V 1J2
Canada

Jones & Bartlett Learning
International
Barb House, Barb Mews
London W6 7PA
United Kingdom

Jones & Bartlett Learning books and products are available through most bookstores and online booksellers. To contact Jones & Bartlett Learning directly, call 800-832-0034, fax 978-443-8000, or visit our website, www.jblearning.com.

The author, editor, and publisher have made every effort to provide accurate information. However, they are not responsible for errors, omissions, or for any outcomes related to the use of the contents of this book and take no responsibility for the use of the products and procedures described. Treatments and side effects described in this book may not be applicable to all people; likewise, some people may require a dose or experience a side effect that is not described herein. Drugs and medical devices are discussed that may have limited availability controlled by the Food and Drug Administration (FDA) for use only in a research study or clinical trial. Research, clinical practice, and government regulations often change the accepted standard in this field. When consideration is being given to use of any drug in the clinical setting, the healthcare provider or reader is responsible for determining FDA status of the drug, reading the package insert, and reviewing prescribing information for the most up-to-date recommendations on dose, precautions, and contraindications, and determining the appropriate usage for the product. This is especially important in the case of drugs that are new or seldom used.

Production Credits

Executive Publisher: Christopher Davis
Editorial Assistant: Sara Cameron
Associate Production Editor: Leah Corrigan
Associate Marketing Manager: Katie Hennessy
Manufacturing and Inventory Control
   Supervisor: Amy Bacus
Composition: Glyph International

Cover Design: Carolyn Downer
Cover Images: (top left) © Thinkstock, (top right) © Monkey Business Images/ ShutterStock, Inc., (bottom) © Yuri Arcurs/ShutterStock, Inc.
Printing and Binding: Malloy, Inc.
Cover Printing: Malloy, Inc.

Library of Congress Cataloging-in-Publication Data
Sheremata, William A.
  100 questions and answers about multiple sclerosis/William A. Sheremata.
—2nd ed.
    p. cm.—(100 questions and answers)
  Includes index.
  ISBN 978-0-7637-8684-7 (alk. paper)
  1. Multiple sclerosis—Miscellanea. 2. Multiple sclerosis—Popular works.
I. Title. II. Title: Hundred and one questions and answers about multiple sclerosis.
  RC377.S55 2011
  616.8'34—dc22
                                                          2010021568
6048

Printed in the United States of America
14 13 12 11 10   10 9 8 7 6 5 4 3 2 1

Contents

Questions 1–15 provide fundamental information about multiple sclerosis (MS):
- What is multiple sclerosis?
- What is a lesion?
- What is white matter?

Questions 16–22 describe common symptoms of multiple sclerosis:
- What are the symptoms of MS? Which symptoms are most common?
- Why am I so fatigued?
- How long do the symptoms of MS last?

Questions 23–37 describe diagnosis, identification, and prognosis of different forms of MS:
- How is a diagnosis of MS made?
- What kinds of MS exist?
- Do all people with MS become disabled?

Questions 38–56 discuss factors that contribute to development of MS:
- Do viruses cause MS?
- What is the role of the immune system in MS?
- Is MS hereditary?

Since the publication of the first edition of *100 Questions & Answers About Multiple Sclerosis,* we have witnessed the diagnosis of multiple sclerosis (MS) in increasing numbers of men and women. Some have concluded that the incidence of MS is increasing. In reality, other factors surely have contributed to this observation. Greater awareness of MS by physicians has led to increased recognition of this illness, especially earlier in its course and in those with milder manifestations of the illness. The once prevalent attitude that less serious problems in MS do not warrant early therapeutic intervention has been dispelled by a number of clinical therapeutic trials. Increasing numbers of neurologists have become aware of the superior therapeutic outcomes seen in drug studies with the early institution of treatment, and they have consequently encouraged their patients to begin treatment at the very outset of illness. As the standard of living increases, there may also be a real increase in the number of patients, because MS occurs predominantly in the middle and upper socioeconomic levels of society.

Astonishing recent advances in both immunology and human genetics have fired the imagination of the public about the possibilities of curing previously incurable diseases. In turn, this awareness has stimulated interest in autoimmune illness and MS in particular. Advanced imaging techniques have also provided new insights into the earliest events in the affected brain, which in turn has stimulated increased interest in early interventions.

Advances in new therapies continue, albeit at a slower pace than the advancement of science. Now we are finally at the brink of the first approvals of new highly effective oral drugs for MS that promise greater benefits as well as ease of use. In this second edition of *100 Questions & Answers About Multiple Sclerosis,* new insights into the factors that contribute to MS and new remedies for MS have been incorporated in the appropriate sections.

In the pretreatment era, MS was the most important cause of chronic disability in young adults, and it occurs more than twice as commonly in women as in men. Ideally, institution of increasingly effective treatment at the earliest possible time will relegate the concern about disability to historical fact.

Multiple sclerosis (MS), a disease with no known cure, begs many more questions than the scientific community can answer. Its origin is unknown, its effects as varied as they are frightening. Those of us living with MS have different ways of dealing with this illness. Our reactions range widely from barely acknowledging our vulnerability (denial), to turning it into a call to arms and our life's mission. (I must admit that I fall into the latter category.) Dr. Sheremata's book, *100 Questions & Answers About Multiple Sclerosis, Second Edition,* attempts to answer the most commonly asked questions that people living with MS—MS survivors, as I call us—have on either end of the spectrum. They include questions that I have asked and tried to answer along my MS journey. I have researched the illness on my own when I did not feel comfortable enough to share my fears with someone wearing a white coat. It took me a while to find patient-friendly physicians who think that no question is too minute, no negative prognosis indisputable. Theirs are the voices I prefer to hear when I am having a particularly bad day and want an explanation about some strange new symptom that has emerged, seemingly from nowhere.

I encourage MS survivors to find healthcare partners who are not only advocates for the illness, but also advocates for them as individuals. Numerous studies show that how patients are diagnosed and their relationships with their healthcare providers influence their ability to manage this illness. *100 Questions & Answers About Multiple Sclerosis, Second Edition,* helps to fill the gap for MS survivors who were diagnosed without compassion or hope, and who don't have open partnerships with their healthcare professionals. Dr. Sheremata adeptly balances his scientific knowledge of the disease and years of clinical practice with an inherent acknowledgment of its emotional impact on patients. He subtly addresses our need to make sense of the inconceivable, offering responses that are thorough, concise, and easily understood by laypeople. (Who needs to be ill and frightened, and to feel too stupid to understand why your body is failing you at the same time—as if this disease does not offer enough sobering experiences on its own.) Additionally, *100 Questions & Answers About Multiple Sclerosis, Second Edition,* recognizes that all of us with MS have shadow patients: those family members, loved ones, friends, and colleagues who live each day with some aspect of this illness, with some part of our new selves under the MonSter, as many of us call MS.

While written for the audience of MS survivors, *100 Questions & Answers About Multiple Sclerosis, Second Edition,* can be an invaluable resource for those who live with us, love us, work with us, and are part of our universe. It helps to explain the strange world of MS, to put the symptoms from the physical to the psychological into perspective, to give them context. As MS continues to extend into "nontraditional" populations, including men, people of color, and even children, I encourage physicians—especially those who are not neurologists by training—to read *100 Questions & Answers About Multiple Sclerosis, Second Edition.* There's no telling when someone will come through their doors with "nonspecific" symptoms and odd episodes and will need to be referred elsewhere.

Montel B. Williams
Founder, The Montel Williams MS Foundation
New York City

For most patients, living with multiple sclerosis (MS) can be frightening, even devastating. Unfortunately, there are many physicians who are so busy that they lose sight of what their patients are experiencing. Especially in this time of managed care, the average practitioner must increase the volume of patient visits to achieve adequate compensation for his or her long investment in medical education, leaving the patient to flounder among often conflicting information without the guidance of a seasoned and caring health provider. In our information age, people are bombarded with much chatter, often far beyond their ability to put it all together in a meaningful way, and all too frequently alarming them about the worst possible outcomes.

The field of neuroimmunology—the science behind MS and its treatment—is becoming constantly more complex. Even busy neurologists usually cannot be conversant with all of the burgeoning knowledge in this field. It thus falls to the academic super-specialist to bridge many branches of science to maintain understanding of advances as they occur.

Dr. Sheremata has brought us, in this small volume, not only many years of ongoing study, but also deep compassion and understanding for the experience of his patients, allowing a firsthand view of what an ideal doctor–patient relationship should be. He has presented the concerns of his patients and demonstrates the actual interaction with them, bringing to bear his extensive experience as an MS expert and his knowledge of the latest achievements in this rapidly progressing field. He inspires confidence and reassurance that there is a light at the end of the tunnel and that his charges are not left without hope. He takes up the difficult task of giving clear and easily understandable explanations to the many questions brought to him. Thus, like the model for the caring physician, Maimonides, Dr. Sheremata has provided a fresh approach that will serve as a guide for the bewildered.

Gerard M. Lehrer, MD

Multiple sclerosis (MS) is a recent illness in the history of human-kind. Although before the latter part of the nineteenth century, several people may have had MS, the first person afflicted with rea-sonable certainty was Sir Augustus d'Este, a grandson of King George III of England. He was born in 1794, 18 years after the American Declaration of Independence. It was through a detailed diary that Douglas Firth recognized the illness and subsequently published extracts from that diary in 1947 (Cambridge University Press). In the mid-nineteenth century in Paris, Jean-Marie Charcot, the first professor of neurology, recognized the cardinal manifesta-tions of MS and the characteristic pathologic changes in the nerv-ous system. In turn, Charcot attributed the recognition of the illness and tissue changes of MS to Cruveilhier, his teacher and the renowned professor of anatomy at the University of Paris. Sigmund Freud, at that time a student under Charcot, became interested in the emotional aspects of MS.

Regardless of who was the first patient affected or who origi-nally described the illness, MS is a uniquely human disease. No comparable natural illness afflicts animals. Experimental models of MS that rely upon diseases produced in animals, such as experi-mental allergic encephalomyelitis (EAE), all fall short for many reasons. For the most part, the study of EAE (as originally intended by scientists) has successfully provided information about immune responses that have been important to human illness, but the specific relevance of EAE to MS has been much more limited.

Important new observations have led to additional insights through the detailed examination of MS brain tissue, especially from those specimens obtained at the very outset of their illness. Studies have confirmed Charcot's original ideas of a central role for myelin in MS. Myelin is a fat-laden tissue that surrounds nerve fibers, allowing them to conduct messages from one nerve cell to another at high speeds. Newer studies, using older and more reliable but more expensive techniques, have shown that extensive myelin damage is commonly present in MS but is often not seen in routine brain magnetic resonance imaging (MRI) scans. The most recent observations, obtained using these older—as well as newer technologies—show that the initial inflammation affects the covering of the brain (the meninges) and then spreads inward into the outer layers of the brain and then into the cortex of the brain; with subsequent involvement of the white matter. The new insights into the earliest events in MS, together with the implementation of newer imaging technology, may lead to even more effective treatment interventions and more effective monitoring of such treatments.

Other studies continue to focus interest on the importance of nerve fiber damage and loss in MS and the development of disability. Additional studies continue to investigate a more newly recognized myelin protein (MOG) as well as the ability of immune reactions to this protein to produce monkey models of disease more closely resembling the human disease MS. One day, these findings may result in a laboratory test that will help confirm the diagnosis at the onset of the illness—a development that has already occurred with the MS-like disease neuromyelitis optica. A specific antibody has been convincingly shown to be both a diagnostic finding and an important factor in that disease. More importantly, these studies collectively are providing new leads as to the cause of MS.

The variety of symptoms and neurologic problems in MS can be bewildering for patients and physicians alike. Compounding this complexity are the emotional reactions of patients with MS to their symptoms. The difficulty in arriving at a diagnosis leads to additional frustration and anxiety for many patients. This is also aggravated by fears (many times unrealistic) of imminent disability. The economic implications of the cost of testing and anticipated loss of income engender concern. The presence of anxiety in patients sometimes prompts them to place undue stress on certain symptoms, all too often leading physicians to conclude that the problem is related to anxiety alone. In my past experience, approximately two of three women ultimately found to have MS were initially diagnosed as being anxious, depressed, or "hysterical." Hopefully, the increasing numbers of patients being diagnosed with MS may reflect greater insight by their physicians, leading to earlier diagnosis.

Many drugs, especially antidepressant and sedative drugs, may affect both symptoms of MS and neurologic functions. Over-the-counter drugs such as dolomite (lithium carbonate), for example, affect both emotional control and immune function. Unfounded claims for a host of substances in health food stores and mail-order sources are legion. The promised benefits may be lacking, but the toxicities of many of these products are real.

Answers to the question "What is MS?" will differ greatly depending on who is asking the question and who is answering. The physician's perspective of MS will depend on his or her education and clinical experience. For instance, a physician's view may reflect the views of scientists who study the changes in normal anatomy and function of the human nervous system. Practicing neurologists may see the question one way when they are trained in general neurology but, when they are trained in the subspecialty of MS, may have quite a different insight. The perspective of the physician trained in psychology or psychiatry may also differ markedly. In the end, all of these views are meaningful to patients and should be integrated for their successful management.

Patients continue to define the question "What is MS?" based on their own particular concerns, which are in a different realm from those of healthcare professionals. Specific patients' concerns are often focused on specific issues. They often emphasize the notion that their symptoms represent a threat to their own physical independence. Their immediate worry is about outcomes of their specific symptoms or limitations of which they may already have become aware. The perspectives of the patient and the physician may intersect later. Often, when the informed patient has his or her original concerns addressed, he or she will then have a better understanding of the scientific underpinnings of the illness and research outcomes as they relate to specific treatment options.

The response to the question "What is MS?" in this book is intended to be meaningful to readers. This question has been addressed from a number of different overlapping perspectives, and asked by a variety of patients with different educational backgrounds and disease manifestations. Many dozens of patients have been asked what their most important question about MS was and which aspects they thought the answer should address. An effort was made to address the specific question they were asking. Many patients were college graduates, whereas others had not graduated from high school. Nevertheless, their questions and concerns were similar. The question "What is multiple sclerosis?" continues to be asked not only by those who submitted their questions for this book but also by the majority of new patients challenged by their new diagnosis.

William A. Sheremata, MD, FRCPC, FACP

This book, *100 Questions & Answers About Multiple Sclerosis, Second Edition*, is dedicated to the many patients who submitted their questions that I have attempted to answer, as well as the many others whom I have served for more than three decades. The questions used in the book were actual questions that patients and their families asked. Many patients asked the same questions, sometimes using different words and coming from different perspectives. The answers are organized in much the same fashion as they are in the other books in the *100 Questions & Answers* series.

The influence of two people on my career must be acknowledged. The first is Norman Geschwind, MD, who was the Putnam Professor of Neurology at Harvard Medical School. This "Renaissance man" inspired me to pursue laboratory research in neuroimmunology as well as clinical training in neurology at the Boston Veterans Affairs Hospital and Boston City Hospital. The second is James Bertrand Cosgrove, MD, of the Montreal Neurological Institute (McGill University). Despite my protests, he took me on as a young faculty member and patiently cultivated my clinical skills, broadening my knowledge of multiple sclerosis.

I am indebted to Karen Miller for her enthusiastic response to my invitation to review, reflect, and comment on the content of this book. I have gotten to know and respect Karen and her husband, David, through interactions in our MS Center. Karen is an exceptionally intelligent, altruistic, and caring woman. With the help of her family, she has accepted her diagnosis and adjusted her life in response to the limitations imposed by MS, interrupting her flourishing and gifted legal career to focus on MS. She participated in a Phase 2 study of Tysabri and became an enthusiastic proponent for the treatment based on her personal experience. Through the years, she has been fortunate to have a loving and supportive family.

The indulgence, patience, and assistance of my own family in completing this book is acknowledged and is deeply appreciated.

William A. Sheremata, MD, FRCPC, FACP

It has been five years since I first provided patient comments for Dr. Sheremata's book, *100 Questions & Answers About Multiple Sclerosis*. I am incredibly humbled by his asking me to participate in the preparation of this book. In my comments for Dr. Sheremata's book and in my testimony before officials from the U.S. Food and Drug Administration regarding Tysabri, I have shared many of my own and my family's private moments and thoughts. When I looked through the current edition of this book, I was tempted to delete everything I had written in the past—in part because I was somewhat surprised at my candor, and in part because I no longer experience some items.

Despite these impulses, I have chosen to leave much of what I wrote for the previous edition untouched, recognizing it as a true expression of an MS patient at a point in time, but also because of the many people who have written that my comments resonated with their own experiences. Some sections I have added or updated because of the inevitable changes due to the nature of MS and my MS in particular, owing to the introduction, removal, and return of Tysabri to my body. Like many patients, my experiences with MS have run the gamut: Physically, I have been a 5.5 on the Extended Disability Scoring System (EDSS) scale and a 1.5 on the EDSS scale. Similarly, I have had a range of emotions—from times when I could not imagine I could cope for one more moment and to times when my joy overcame the MS. I am grateful for how fortunate I am to have my doctors, my family, my friends, and my faith.

In the sixteenth century, Michel de Montaigne wrote, "Many things that I would not want to tell anyone, I tell the public; and for my most secret knowledge and thoughts I send my most faithful friends to the bookseller's shop." Today, in the twenty-first century, I write similarly, and I hope that my candor is of help to someone, somehow.

Karen Miller

PART ONE

The Basics

What is multiple sclerosis?

What is a lesion?

What is white matter?

More . . .

1. What is multiple sclerosis?

In the classic sense, multiple sclerosis (MS) is a disease of the **central nervous system** (**CNS**: the brain and spinal cord) that most commonly affects young adults. *Sclerosis* means "hardening"; *multiple sclerosis* means that there are multiple areas of hardened tissue in the brain and spinal cord due to scarring. The word *disease* means a loss of a feeling of ease (i.e., "dis-ease") or, otherwise stated, a loss of a sense of well-being. This is a meaningful definition for MS patients faced with a bewildering variety of other specific symptoms. Often, patients afflicted with MS have difficulty describing just how they feel. Although the MS patient appreciates and understands this concept, many healthy persons, including physicians, family members, and friends, unfortunately, often do not.

The **neurologist** recognizes MS as a disease with many different symptoms that come and go, affecting different parts of the nervous system. To be considered as a manifestation of MS (an attack), a symptom should last at least 1 day (24 hours). Any of the presenting problems of MS may appear singly or in combination. Some of the symptoms can be evidence of other illnesses unrelated to MS.

The question "What is MS?" is like the proverbial blind men and the elephant: The description depends on the individual experience. The following questions have been arranged to help you build a working knowledge of what this illness is.

Karen's comment:

My MS is my MS. Each person who has MS has different symptoms, different manifestations of the same symptom, and different ways of dealing with (or not) the illness. I do

Central nervous system (CNS)

The brain and spinal cord.

Neurologist

A physician specializing in the diagnosis and care of neurological disease.

To be considered as a manifestation of MS (an attack), a symptom should last at least 1 day (24 hours).

not claim to know what is best for anyone else with MS. Indeed, many times I am not certain even for myself. Unlike what MS is, I do have a sense of what MS is not. For me, MS is not a blessing. MS is not a curse. MS is not my fault. MS is not something that anyone could have prevented, and MS is not an excuse. Perhaps, most importantly, MS is not the end of my ability to live and to love.

2. Where does MS occur in the nervous system?

All of the symptoms and abnormalities that neurologists find during the neurologic examination, and that are thought to be evidence of MS, are the result of **lesions** of the brain and, more often, lesions of the spinal cord. The loss of well-being is probably the consequence of the **immune system** becoming activated.

3. What is a lesion?

Physicians often use the term "lesion" to indicate focal tissue damage in some part of the body. MS symptoms that neurologists are "tuned into" are the consequence of **inflammation** in different areas of the nervous system. Inflammation occurs in spots that are scattered in the brain and spinal cord, called **plaques**. If these plaques are large enough, they usually show up in brain or spinal cord **magnetic resonance imaging (MRI)** scans. Nevertheless, most brain lesions do not cause symptoms, although it is true that a large volume of brain lesions is more likely to be associated with cognitive problems, particularly with memory.

4. What is a plaque?

Spots of inflammation and scarring that are responsible for the hardening in the brain and spinal cord are often called plaques. They are called plaques because

Lesion

A localized area of tissue damage, or pathology, of any cause.

Immune system

The host defense against infection, which consists of the white blood cells (leukocytes), including lymphocytes and monocytes circulating in the blood and other tissues (including the bone marrow), lymph nodes, and the thymus.

Inflammation

The accumulation of fluid, plasma proteins, and white blood cells initiated by physical injury, infection, or local immune response.

Plaques

The plate-like hardened areas of myelin damage and scarring in MS, which are located in the brain and spinal cord.

Magnetic resonance imaging (MRI)

Imaging of the brain or other organs obtained by the use of magnetic fields and radio frequency together with computerized tomography.

The Basics

Optic nerve

The second cranial nerve, which is actually an extension of the brain. Nerve fibers from the retina travel to the brain through the optic nerve.

Cerebral cortex

The layer of neurons covering the entire outside surface of the brain. It appears gray as compared with the white matter inside the brain.

Gray matter

The cortex of the brain; the outermost layer of the brain that is made up of neurons. It completely covers the white matter. The neurons in the cortex send nerve fibers to, and receive them from, other parts of the brain and spinal cord.

Neuron

Nerve cell; the morphologic and functional unit of the nervous system. It consists of the nerve cell body, the dendrite, and the axon.

they looked like little plates to Charcot, the French doctor who first found them more than a century ago. *Plaque* is the French word for "plate." Plaques may also occur in the **optic nerve**, which is actually part of brain and not really a "nerve."

5. *What is white matter?*

The outermost layer of the brain is called the **cerebral cortex,** or **gray matter**, and is made up of brain cells (**neurons**). The cortex completely covers the **white matter**, which makes up the largest part of the brain and serves to connect different neurons. The neurons in the cortex send nerve fibers (**axons**) to and receive axons from other parts of the brain and spinal cord. Nerve fibers covered with **myelin** can be found within the cortex as well.

White matter is largely made of myelin. It gets its name because it contains a lot of fat and has a whitish appearance. MRI scans actually show areas of increased water content in the brain, which indicate areas of inflammation or scarring from previous damage. These areas of damage may be either plaques caused by MS or the result of some other disease process. It has recently been suggested that damage to myelin that is not caused by inflammation will not show up in an ordinary MRI brain scan (see **Figures 1** and **2**).

Recent research has shown that the first signs of inflammation actually begin in the coverings of the brain (the meninges) and then spread into the outermost parts of the cortex. Actual plaques may form inside the cortex, with the "typical" lesions being found in the white matter only later in the disease process. Although this kind of spread may occur only in the occasional and most severely affected patients (and is confirmed through brain biopsies), this finding may explain complaints

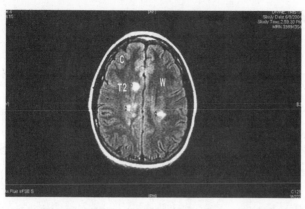

Figure 1 MRI of the brain. A transverse section shows "T2" bright spots in the white matter (labeled "W") of the brain. Note the cortex ("C"), the slightly gray area in the image, which is the layer over the white matter. The bright T2 areas are often referred to by physicians as "hyperintense areas of T2 signal" and at other times are simply called plaques.

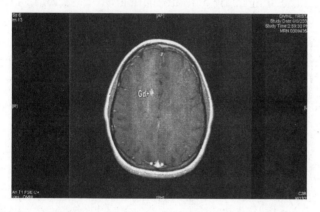

Figure 2 MRI of the same brain shown in Figure 1. A transverse section shows a smaller bright area labeled "Gd+" in a different type of MRI. This is a "T1 weighted" image with an "enhancing" lesion that appeared after gadolinium was injected intravenously. The areas that were bright in Figure 1 are not bright in this image. The enhancing lesion is evidence of active inflammation present at the time of the MRI scan. Note that the enhancing lesion is a small portion of one of the T2 lesions shown in Figure 1. This means that only part of the bright area in Figure 1 is "active" and is added onto a pre-existing plaque.

White matter

A part of the brain largely made of myelin. It gets its name because it contains a lot of fat and looks whitish compared to the cortex.

Axon

A nerve fiber arising from a neuron (nerve cell). Signals (messages) arising from one neuron are transmitted to another via the axon.

Myelin

Lipoproteinaceous material composed of alternating layers of lipid and protein of the myelin sheath.

The Basics

of memory and other cognitive complaints that some patients have.

Axons are damaged by the inflammatory process associated with MS, and some are lost permanently. This loss of axons is thought to be important in the development of disability and disease progression.

6. What is myelin?

Nerve fibers (axons) coming from neurons and going to connect with other neurons are surrounded by myelin. The axons and the myelin that cover them make up the white matter. Myelin insulates the nerve fibers, just like the insulation found on copper wires. The insulation provided by the myelin sheath is important because it greatly speeds up the communication between different areas of the brain and reduces the energy required to transmit messages. Amazingly, myelin allows a signal to travel the length of a football field in 1 second. The plaques formed as a result of inflammation are areas of damage to myelin and, therefore, interfere with the ability of axons to send messages. Although symptoms of MS will depend on the location of the plaque, many plaques in the brain will not cause any obvious neurologic symptoms (**Figure 3**).

7. What are "oligos?"

Cell

The smallest unit of a living animal. Cells are enclosed in a membrane (the cell membrane). They have a nucleus containing chromosomes, mitochondria, and other "machinery."

Oligodendrocyte

A type of glial cell that gives rise to the myelin sheath. Each cell forms several myelin sheaths.

Myelin on the nerve fibers (axons) is arranged like beads on a necklace. The **cells** that make myelin are called **oligodendrocytes** (also known as "oligos"). Each of these oligodendrocytes sends up to two dozen tentacle-like arms to jelly-roll-like nodes of myelin separated by little gaps. Myelin is very important because it helps the nerve fibers save 99% of the energy that they would otherwise have to expend to transmit signals. Damage to myelin alone results in messages becoming blocked at the site of damage. Inflammation itself can also damage the nerve fiber directly, although there is probably always accompanying myelin damage. Recovery from an attack of MS—at least early recovery—is

The Basics

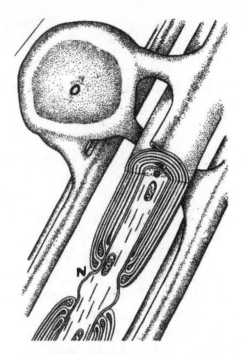

Figure 3 An oligodendrocyte is labeled as "O" in the upper left of the drawing. Three of many arm-like extensions of the cell are shown in this drawing. Each of these extensions wrap around separate areas of individual axons, forming myelin sheaths. The myelin sheath is cut away (labeled as N) showing a bulging bit of axon between two myelin sheaths.

Source: *Neurobiology*, G.M. Shepherd. Oxford University Press, Inc.

probably the result of inflammation subsiding. Repair to the axon and myelin may occur within limits.

Over the last half century, neuropathologists ranging from Dr. Raymond Adams at Harvard University to Dr. John Prineas in Australia have interpreted changes in the brain as showing an initial insult to oligodendrocytes. Others, notably Dr. Peter Lampert, have used serial brain sections to convincingly show that each plaque in the entire brain of every brain studied is associated with a tiny blood vessel (a venule) in the middle. This finding is important because it shows that the offending agent (cells and/or antibodies) comes from the blood. This understanding is basic to virtually all

White blood cells

Leukocytes of the blood. A general term used for all white blood cells, including lymphocytes, poly-morphonuclear leukocytes, and monocytes.

Lymphocytes

White blood cells (B cells and T cells); part of the immune system.

Monocyte

A leukocyte (white blood cell). Mono-cytes are part of the human body's immune system; they protect the body against infections and move quickly to sites of infection.

Macrophages

Monocytes from the bloodstream that have been "turned on" by interacting with lymphocytes.

Antibody

Proteins made by the immune system that defend the body against infectious agents. At times, antibody may be directed against the body's own tissues, resulting in autoim-mune disease. Anti-body is produced when B cells are stim-ulated by antigen.

of the effective treatments for prevention of attacks and disability in MS.

8. What causes the inflammation in the plaque?

Inflammation in the nervous system is usually caused by **white blood cells** (WBCs), called **lymphocytes** (mostly CD4+ cells); **monocytes** (**macrophages**) from the bloodstream usually cause inflammation in the nervous system. Cells and fluids in the blood are normally restricted from entering the nervous system by the blood–brain barrier. This barrier is formed by endothelial cells lining the venules with "tight junctions," uniquely occurring in the brain and spinal cord. A second layer of "foot processes" from astrocytes (star-like cells) in the brain and spinal cord buttresses this barrier. In the process of inflammation, these WBCs eat holes through the lining of the smallest blood vessels (venules) and enter the nervous system. Lymphocytes and macrophages are not normally present in the nervous system.

In some patients, a different type of immune reaction occurs in which **antibody** plays an important role in damaging myelin. In some individuals, antibody may be the sole cause of myelin damage. In another group of patients with a different variation of MS, antibody damage may lead to additional damage caused by another kind of lymphocyte (CD8+ cells). Despite this possibility, in ordinary cases of MS, it is not yet clear how common or important CD8-mediated damage is.

9. What is a macrophage?

Macrophages (meaning "big eaters") are actually monocytes from the bloodstream that have been "turned on" by interacting with lymphocytes, which themselves have been turned on by other macrophages that have encountered a foreign protein. Recent research has emphasized the role that these cells play in producing damage in MS. They can be activated by a large number of different mechanisms. Macrophages have an amazing appetite and ability to damage tissue. For example, in **tuberculosis**, macrophages cause the tissue damage to lungs and other tissues. It is clear that certain cells (so-called microglial cells) in the brain are capable of performing the same functions in the nervous system as macrophages do in the bloodstream. They are included as part of the conceptualized "innate" immune system in the nervous system. New emphasis is being placed on the role of this innate immune system in MS.

In MS, as seen in **Figures 4** and **5**, macrophages appear to be the primary cause of myelin damage. Using an

Tuberculosis

The disease that results from infection by *Mycobacterium tuberculosis*. Although this disease most commonly affects the lungs, any tissue in the body can be involved.

The Basics

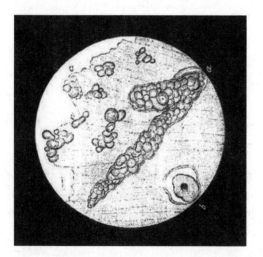

Figure 4   A drawing of a plaque by Charcot using a simple microscope. Charcot described the illustration as "Patch of sclerosis in the fresh state. Lymphatic sheath of a vessel distended by voluminous fatty globules." The fat-laden cells are surrounding a tiny blood vessel in an MS plaque and the cells are filled with myelin. These cells are actually macrophages that have damaged myelin, resulting in "demyelination."

Source: JM Charcot. The diseases of the nervous system. (The new Sydenham Society London, translation by G. Sigerson). 1867. p178: Fig. 10.

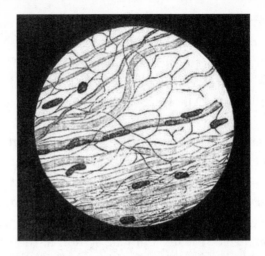

Figure 5   Another drawing by Charcot showing loss of normal myelin around a small blood vessel. This blood vessel is a venule with five or six long, bean-like nuclei oriented more or less horizontally in the middle of the drawing. Also seen are spaghetti-like axons without myelin, which appear smaller than the other axons with their myelin intact. This observation led to multiple sclerosis being termed as a "demyelinating disease."

Source: JM Charcot. The diseases of the nervous system. (The new Sydenham Society London, translation by G. Sigerson). 1867. p173: Fig. 9.

electron microscope, you can see actual chunks of myelin inside macrophages in plaques.

10. How do the white blood cells get into the brain and spinal cord?

Molecule

A very small mass of matter; the smallest amount of a substance that can exist alone, which must consist of at least two atoms.

Adhesion molecules

Velcro-like proteins on the surface of white blood cells and other cells that allow them to stick to the lining of veins.

When lymphocytes become turned on by an immune reaction, they, in turn, "turn on" or "activate" blood monocytes. Once activated, monocytes become macrophages and develop incredible appetites. The activated lymphocytes and macrophages have "Velcro-like" **molecules** on them called **adhesion molecules**, which are specifically termed as "selectins" or "integrins." These cells stick to the inside of the tiniest blood vessels that have corresponding adhesion molecules; they then become able to eat their way through the vessel into the nervous system (**Figure 6**).

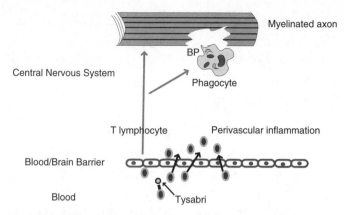

Figure 6   Immunopathogenesis of MS. Mechanisms of demyelination are shown diagrammatically in this illustration. Cells (lymphocytes and macrophages) cross the blood–brain barrier and enter the brain and spinal cord (the central nervous system). These cells then damage myelin. Myelin antibody may also play some role in demyelination. MBP is a major protein component of myelin; Tysabri stops these cells from attaching to the cerebral endothelium and crossing. Note the tight junctions of the endothelium.

11. Can inflammation and plaques be stopped?

Treatment can reduce or even prevent inflammation. For example, **adrenocorticotrophic hormone (ACTH)**; Acthar Gel, **steroids**, and certain other drugs may be used to stop or reverse inflammation. These drugs work in a number of different ways (i.e., they have a number of different actions) that contribute to this end. The use of these drugs is discussed in the section dealing with treatment. "**ABC**" (Avonex, Betaseron, and Copaxone) therapy, Tysabri, and the new oral agents for MS are addressed there.

12. At what age do people get MS?

MS has been described as the most common illness causing disability in people younger than the age of 45 years. Most people, especially women, have their first symptoms and are diagnosed before the age of 30 years.

Adrenocorticotrophic hormone (ACTH)

A hormone made in the brain and stored in the pituitary gland at the base of the brain. It is the only Food and Drug Administration (FDA)-approved treatment for shortening MS attacks. Also called corticotrophin.

Steroids

A large family of chemical substances, including many hormones, that are chemically defined as containing a tetracyclic cyclopenta alpha phenanthrene skeleton.

"ABC"

A commonly used unofficial reference to Avonex, Betaseron, and Copaxone, all of which are approved drugs for MS treatment.

The Basics

However, one in every five MS patients will have onset of the illness and will be diagnosed *after* the age of 45 years. This is equally true from the west coast of Canada to south Florida.

13. Do women get MS more often than men?

Women do get MS more often than men.

Yes, women do get MS more often than men. Approximately 70% of all patients diagnosed with MS are women (all the way from western Canada to the southeastern part of the United States). This difference in gender-based rates is even more pronounced in patients younger than the age of 30 years. Almost four of every five persons with onset of illness before the age of 30 years will be women. In contrast, the onset of MS after the age of 40 years is slightly more common in men.

Demyelinating disease

Disease primarily associated with damage to (demyelination of) myelin, such as acute disseminated encephalomyelitis and MS.

Hormone

The internal secretion of an endocrine organ such as the adrenal glands or ovaries. Hormones are important chemical messengers that communicate with distant organs in the body.

Estrogen

The steroid produced by the ovary that is responsible for the secondary sexual characteristics of adult females.

The reason for MS occurring more frequently in women than in men is unknown. Female experimental animals develop **demyelinating disease** more predictably and of greater severity than males. This finding and the fact that women have decreased disease activity during pregnancy suggest that sex **hormones** influence disease activity. The finding that a placental **estrogen** (a hormone) has a favorable effect in women with MS supports this theory. The administration of this oral estrogen prevented new active brain lesions in a recent MRI study and is currently undergoing further investigation.

14. Does MS affect people of different races differently?

Most of the people with MS are of European descent. MS is less common in African Americans (about half as common) and appears to be even less common among

Asians living in the United States. These observations are in agreement with the finding that MS is rare in Africa and in Asia. Nevertheless, in Australia—a country that is populated predominantly by people of European descent—MS is less common than in the United States, Canada, and Europe. Also, a "north–south gradient" (explained in Question 15) is apparently seen in Australia.

15. How does latitude affect MS?

Observations that MS is more common in the northern latitudes of Europe and North America were originally interpreted as showing a latitude effect, the so-called north–south gradient. Recent evidence suggests that this effect may be an artifact reflecting immigration patterns. Emigrating northern (European) people originally settled in the northern latitudes in America that more closely resembled their homelands. It has been found that veterans (in U.S. studies) with Scandinavian surnames living in the northern United States have the same risk of MS as those who live in the South. In the past, few neurologists lived in the southern United States. In fact, the author's clinic in Miami was the first in the southeastern United States to have a full-time staff devoted to MS patients. Many areas of Australia also lack neurologists. Because a diagnosis of MS is not accepted unless made by a neurologist, the diagnosis is obviously made less commonly in under-served areas such as northern Australia and, at least in the past, in the southern United States.

Recently, there have been attempts to correlate greater sun exposure, and therefore higher vitamin D levels, with a reduced risk of MS. While new evidence points to an important linkage of higher vitamin D levels with a lower risk of MS (and hence a correlation of

MS incidence with latitude), problems arise when trying to prove this relationship. Heat exposure brings out symptoms in MS, which prompts patients to avoid the sun in hot climates. Indeed, serum vitamin D levels in Florida MS patients are most often quite low. This may have been important in the past but it does not seem to be relevant at present.

PART TWO

Symptoms of Multiple Sclerosis

What are the symptoms of MS? Which symptoms are most common?

Why am I so fatigued?

How long do the symptoms of MS last?

More . . .

16. What are the symptoms of MS? Which symptoms are most common?

Symptoms of MS vary from common problems such as unexplained difficulty in walking (occurring in about half of patients at the very beginning) to relatively less common problems, such as blurred vision, to truly uncommon symptoms, such as repeated sudden and brief spasms in one or more limbs (paroxysmal **dystonia**).

Despite the many different medical problems that can cause walking difficulty, the experienced neurologist assumes that a young person using a cane most likely has MS. Also, when someone is diagnosed with **optic neuritis** (or **retrobulbar neuritis**), we know that the vast majority of patients will be diagnosed with MS within 15 years. Approximately half of those affected by optic neuritis will have another episode of neurologic difficulty within a year. If they see an experienced neurologist, they will then be diagnosed with "clinically definite MS."

There are so many different symptoms of MS that it is almost meaningless to list them. Nevertheless, almost all of these difficulties can occur in other neurologic diseases. It is the relapsing–remitting character of symptoms that serves as the best evidence that any particular neurologic manifestation is caused by MS. The appearance of neurologic problems such as difficulty in walking (i.e., the "attack") followed by improvement (i.e., the "remission") is what characterizes MS in the typical patient.

Although a neurologist is required to make a diagnosis of MS, confirming this diagnosis may be difficult in some patients. In the past, the diagnosis of MS was

Dystonia

Abnormal muscle tone usually resulting in an abnormal position (posture) relative to the rest of the body.

Optic neuritis (retrobulbar neuritis)

An inflammation of the optic nerve that is characterized by pain and variable loss of vision. Most patients who develop this condition will eventually be diagnosed as having MS.

usually delayed for many years. Two decades ago, the typical delay in diagnosis in the United States was 7 years or more; in the United Kingdom, it was as long as 11 years. This kind of delay should not happen in this day and age.

Difficulty in walking is the most commonly recognized difficulty in MS when patients are first seen by a physician. It occurs in approximately half of all patients at the outset of their illness. This problem is often due to mild weakness or stiffness of one leg, although sometimes both legs are affected. It is rather common to have the difficulty appear during more prolonged physical activity and particularly with heat exposure. Both of these conditions raise body temperature and bring out symptoms in MS. Balance problems may also present as gait difficulty.

Difficulty in walking is the most commonly recognized difficulty in MS when patients are first seen by a physician.

Actually, numbness and tingling in one or both hands or feet are probably the most common symptoms in the early stages of MS. However, the patient or the physician may not seriously consider them as evidence of illness without other accompanying symptoms. It is general knowledge that otherwise normal people may occasionally have these transient symptoms. A neurologist should determine if numbness or tingling, with or without any other symptom, lasts a full day or longer. Recurrent numbness over a period of time is of equal importance.

Difficulties with coordination or the appearance of **tremor** should always be considered to be evidence of nervous system disease and should be investigated. In the past, some neurologists would not make a diagnosis of MS without the presence of tremor, shaky eyes (**nystagmus**), and difficulty in speaking, which are

Tremor

An oscillating rhythmic movement usually involving an extremity. Head movement may accompany tremor but is termed titubation.

Nystagmus

Fine rhythmic oscillating movements of the eyeball.

Charcot's triad

A collection of symptoms, including nystagmus (shaky eyes), dysarthria, and tremor (slurred speech and shaking of the hands and body) that was described as being characteristic of MS. Although it does occur in MS, it is rare.

Glaucoma

A disease of the eye characterized by increased intraocular pressure causing damage to the retina and impaired vision.

Trigeminal neuralgia

Intense, brief, facial pain typically occurring on one side. It is uncommon before 65 years of age, except in MS. Its occurrence in young adults is usually a sign of MS.

collectively known as **Charcot's triad**. In reality, only a minority of patients ever develop all three of these symptoms; when they are present simultaneously, it signals the presence of particularly severe disease.

Although visual problems are less common at onset of illness, they become relatively common over the lifetime of patients with untreated MS. A physician should always evaluate visual symptoms, especially double vision or blurring of vision accompanied by pain in one or both eyes. MS-caused blindness is uncommon. **Glaucoma** is a more common cause of blindness.

Karen's comment:

When I am asked how I am, "I have MS" seems to be the best answer. To go into details feels—as one person put it— like "Aunt Bertha's bunions": a bit boring, a bit graphic, and at times a bit scary. With that caveat, I provide more information here.

*When I thought I had a problem with a tooth, it turned out to be MS. It took the dentist, an x-ray, and my sister's research about **trigeminal neuralgia** to convince me that the overwhelming pain in my face was MS. When I had a tightness in my chest, it turned out to be MS. It took a heart specialist, my wearing a heart monitor, and several heart exams to reassure my neurologist and my husband that the extra heartbeats were MS. When I temporarily lost my vision, it turned out to be MS. When I forgot what year it was, it turned out to be MS . . . and so on.*

Sometimes a symptom may not be MS per se but rather a physical difficulty made worse or unusual because of the MS. Even things that previously were not a problem can have an effect. For example, after 51 years of using generic bandages, going to the dentist, and wearing rubber gloves at home, I developed an allergy to latex. Many people without MS do also. Unfortunately, because of the MS, my immune system reacted so strongly to a brief touch on my cheek by a dental assistant that the new allergy caused my face to swell and one eye to close. As a result, I had to be seen on an urgent basis by a dermatologist who specializes in infectious disease and I missed the high school graduation of one of my beloved nieces. I compounded the situation with treatments that I became allergic to and by crying. Eventually, the dermatologist discovered the latex allergy, and in a few days I was fine. We have pictures commemorating my face in Cyclops mode— and more importantly, pictures of my niece's graduation.

If I have a new medical problem, it is appropriate to rule out non-MS causes. Sometimes a sore tooth, extra heartbeats, blurry vision, memory lapses, skin growths, and a raspy throat are what they would be for someone without MS. However, more often than not, the new (and sometimes weird) symptom can be traced to a brain, nerve, or muscle cell that fires, misfires, or stops firing because of MS. With approximately 10 billion brain cells, 45 miles of nerves, and 650 muscles, if something is wrong with me, the odds are that it is MS.

17. Why am I so fatigued?

Fatigue (a lack of energy) is a common and important manifestation of MS and is even more common than numbness and tingling. Although not specific to MS, it occurs in the vast majority of patients. Qualitatively, it is not possible to state that the fatigue is different in patients with MS than in persons with "chronic fatigue syndrome." Many MS patients report that it is their major problem. Increased fatigue accompanies most attacks of MS and is an important factor aggravating other manifestations of MS. In actuality, when many patients complain of "fatigue," they often are referring

Fatigue
A type of tiredness that is different from drowsiness. Drowsiness is feeling the need to sleep, whereas fatigue is a lack of energy and motivation. Apathy (a feeling of indifference or not caring about what happens) and drowsiness can be symptoms of fatigue.

19

Fatigability

The loss of muscle strength following repeated use or testing of one or more muscles.

Infectious mononucleosis

Glandular fever. It is a common form of infection with the Epstein-Barr virus (EBV) and is characterized by fever, fatigue, and enlarged lymph nodes, often accompanied by rash, splenic enlargement, and hepatic enzyme elevation.

to **fatigability**. A typical example of this occurs when an individual begins walking without difficulty, but after a hundred yards or so must either hold onto another person or object or must stop. Many patients run out of energy by midday and must stop and rest. An unexplained severe lack of energy often precedes other symptoms associated with the onset of an attack of MS.

To put this symptom in perspective, everyone experiences fatigue and physical activity normally induces fatigue. In MS, however, fatigue is a frequent complicating symptom (perhaps the most common symptom of MS) and can be overwhelming. This type of fatigue occurs during attacks of illness, and it may even precede attacks. Sometimes it lasts for long periods of time and may be diagnosed as chronic fatigue syndrome. Patients who have had viral hepatitis or **infectious mononucleosis** in the past state that the fatigue they experienced then is the same severe fatigue accompanying MS. Whereas patients with infectious mononucleosis and hepatitis recover eventually, those with MS are subject to persistence or recurrences for the remainder of their lives. The more effective the treatment (discussed in Part 6, Treatment of Multiple Sclerosis), the more likely the sense of well-being is to return.

Most physicians, including neurologists, find it difficult or impossible to assess fatigue. To compensate for this problem, scoring systems for quantifying this complaint have been developed to help evaluate its response to treatment. A few physicians in MS centers use these "fatigue scales," but others reject them as being "too subjective." Fatigue responds to certain drugs; in contrast, "fatigability" often imposes physical limitations and requires pacing of physical activity. It is important to distinguish these terms because "fatigue," as defined by the Social Security Administration, is actually fatigability and is a criterion for the evaluation of disability. The proper use of the **Extended Disability Scoring System (EDSS)** by a neurologist experienced in its use is a valid way of evaluating "fatigue" (fatigability).

18. How long do the symptoms of MS last?

To be considered a symptom of MS, the symptom should last at least 24 hours. However, certain rare symptoms, such as recurrent brief spasms in one or more limbs (paroxysmal dystonia), can be recognized as part of MS. Although they are of short duration, typically seconds to minutes, they are identified because they recur in a stereotyped fashion. Other symptoms, such as the loss of muscle tone, difficulty with articulation during speaking, pain, and so on, may be due to MS as well. Unfortunately, these manifestations are unfamiliar to most non-MS doctors and are likely to be attributed to emotional problems.

Symptoms in MS typically develop over a period of several days but rarely evolve over more than 2 or 3 weeks. They typically dissipate over a much longer period of time than when they initially appeared, often over a period of weeks and sometimes months. Rest certainly shortens the duration of symptoms. Before the advent of ACTH treatment for MS more than a half a century ago, rest was the only effective treatment, as it was in tuberculosis since the days of Hippocrates in ancient Greece.

Karen's comment:

How long do the symptoms of MS last? Too long! Closely correlated with the maxim, "If it is a symptom, it is probably MS," is the notion, "If it is an MS symptom, it is not necessarily new." I have had certain symptoms last a few

Extended Disability Scoring System (EDSS)

A grading scale for recording levels of neurologic disability, which was originally developed by Kurtzke. It is used universally for recording disability.

Symptoms of Multiple Sclerosis

days and some have lasted for 6 months. When I ask myself how I am, or as some have phrased it, "take inventory," I am torn between focusing on and ignoring each symptom, variation of a symptom, manifestation of a symptom, manifestation of a variation of a symptom, and so on. Independent of a particular symptom, what does not go away is the MS itself. Like other chronic illnesses, it is just that—chronic. There are no days off. Ultimately it is all MS for better and for worse, and until there is a cure—forever.

19. Is my stuttering due to my MS?

Stuttering is not part of MS. However, intermittent difficulty with speech that somewhat resembles stuttering (paroxysmal **dysarthria**) was recognized as a rare manifestation of MS 40 years ago. This difficulty with articulation is often associated with difficulty in finding the "right" word. It is rarely recognized as a manifestation of MS, and many doctors incorrectly regard it as an emotional problem. Misdiagnosis is unfortunate, because this disorder is amenable to treatment.

Dysarthria
Slurred speech.

A number of other brief (typically lasting seconds to minutes), recurrent stereotyped paroxysmal (short duration) manifestations rarely accompany MS. Sometimes they are mistaken as **seizures**, but fortunately they respond to anticonvulsant (antiseizure) treatment as if they were seizures. However, they do not require lifelong drug therapy but rather long-term (3 to 6 months) treatment. These manifestations of MS usually respond to lower doses of drugs—doses that would not control seizures. Tegretol (carbamazepine) is effective in small doses (1/2 tablet 3 to 4 times daily). The drug is well tolerated, is relatively inexpensive, and is the drug of choice in my practice. It is beyond the scope of this book to discuss these issues further.

Seizure
An epileptic event consisting of loss of consciousness usually associated with tonic and/or clonic movements.

22

20. How severe are attacks of MS?

The manifestations of MS are often mild and transient but less commonly may be severe. Both patients and physicians often think of MS attacks as lasting for weeks. However, in a recently published study where both the patient and the examiner were "blinded"—that is, neither knew which treatment was being administered (i.e., a double-blind study)—we found that most attacks lasted only 5 to 7 days before resolving spontaneously (without active treatment).

Shortly after the discovery of MS as a disease in Paris; Uhthoff, a Viennese physician, found that increases in body temperature could temporarily result in blurred vision in a young man who had recovered from an attack of optic neuritis. This ("Uhthoff") phenomenon can also result in other symptoms occurring transiently (or as long as body temperature is increased). It is important to recognize that these increases in symptoms brought out by elevated body temperature are *not* attacks of MS. If the same symptoms occur in the absence of a fever or elevated body temperature and last a day or longer, however, they may be mild attacks of MS.

Attacks of MS can sometimes be severe and require a prolonged period of recovery, sometimes lasting as long as a year or so, but this is unusual. ACTH and high-dose intravenous (IV) steroids shorten the period of recovery. Nevertheless, many attacks (the majority) are mild, and treatment is not needed. Fortunately, effective treatments for MS (see the section of this book discussing treatment) reduce the risk of these severe attacks more than the risk of milder attacks. In the studies that led to its approval by the U.S. Food and Drug Administration (FDA), one type of **interferon**, known as interferon-beta, reduced the frequency of severe attacks by almost

The manifestations of MS are often mild and transient but less commonly may be severe.

Interferons

Cytokines; proteins made by lymphocytes that can induce cells to resist viral replication.

Symptoms of Multiple Sclerosis

50% as compared with a 30% reduction in overall actions. This difference becomes more meaningful when you realize that severe attacks are associated with an inability to function and are usually treated in hospital.

Karen's comment:

This question is perhaps best answered at the end of an attack. While it is going on, it may seem severe. Or if it is a new symptom, it can be jolting when something I thought would work does not. If the effects go away, then I am less likely to label the attack as "severe." I have not had an attack that I knew would get better while it was occurring.

Some of my symptoms have lasted a few days, and some have lasted for 6 months. I have had periods when I was unable to walk, to swallow easily, and/or to see. The symptom that has resolved eventually and that I have had last the longest and found most limiting is vertigo.

When I moved in certain ways or people and objects moved, it triggered severe dizziness, the room spinning, me feeling like I was spinning, and accompanying nausea. The banners on a TV screen, cars on the road, ceiling fans, and my husband moving his fork at dinner are examples of what I had to avoid seeing. Thus I stayed indoors. I listened to recorded books. I ate meals next to, rather than across, from my husband—all compensatory processes. As time went on, the accidental triggers occurred less, but the points at which I felt I could not live with the vertigo occurred more. The vertigo started suddenly and ended quickly. Eight months later, I felt dizzy again. I sobbed, thinking that I was going to have another long bout, but it turned out to be just the flu. When I did have the next episode of vertigo, I thought it would never end. However, like many symptoms, with time, it did.

21. Can I go blind with MS?

Although visual loss accompanying attacks of MS, diagnosed as optic neuritis or retrobulbar neuritis, may occasionally be severe, blindness is unusual. There may be a small blind spot left after an attack; occasionally, this may be large enough to interfere with vision. There is no convincing evidence that any form of treatment reduces the risk of significant residual visual impairment. Glaucoma, which is another type of eye disease and is unrelated to MS, is more common as a cause of blindness in MS patients.

Karen's comment:

My vision problems range from a bit of blurriness to a complete lack of sight. I inherited extreme **myopia***; I wear contact lenses and glasses even in the shower. Before MS, changes in my vision required new prescriptions and picking out the least offensive frames. MS vision symptoms and optic neuritis were entirely new and different experiences for me. I was unaware of my visual field shrinking until Dr. Allen, the* **ophthalmologist** *who has seen me since I was age 9, noted this condition, and Dr. Byron Lam, the neuro-ophthalmologist at Bascom Palmer Eye Institute, confirmed it. MS eye problems can be caused by how the MS affects the optic nerve, the eye muscles, and the eyelid muscles. Tysabri and yoga exercises have improved some of my vision deficits.*

The first time I lost my vision, I panicked, certain that it would not return. The second time, I panicked less. The third time, my family worried less. The fourth time, I nonchalantly said to myself, "Oh, it's just MS, and I've done this before," but I was not entirely reassured. Each time, I was very relieved and a bit surprised when my vision returned.

Myopia

Short-sightedness.

Ophthalmologist

A physician who specializes in the diagnosis and treatment of diseases of the eye.

22. What causes walking difficulty in MS?

Difficulty with walking in MS can result from plaques in different places in the brain stem and spinal cord. The location of the plaques determines, in large part, whether that difficulty is due to the particular problems of weakness, loss of sensation, or incoordination of the legs. In certain places in the brain and spinal cord, plaques can produce weakness; those in the back part of the spinal cord cause certain kinds of sensation loss (position sense); others in the **cerebellum** and its connections lead to incoordination in the legs. Any or all of these disturbances can contribute to gait difficulty.

The most common complaint associated with difficulty in walking is "weakness." When a patient complains of "weakness," he or she is often describing one of several different problems. Muscle weakness in nervous system disease is often the result of messages not getting to the muscles from the brain and spinal cord. A signal or message may begin in the brain (the precentral or motor area of the brain), but it has to travel to neurons located in the spinal cord, perhaps as far as 3 feet away. The signal travels down a small part of the spinal cord called the pyramidal tract. One or more MS plaques along the way may prevent part, or all, of that message from getting to the neuron, resulting in "weakness" and difficulty standing and walking. The larger the plaque, the more likely it is to interfere with many messages to many neurons and produce more weakness of the muscles that these neurons supply.

Sometimes patients complain of weakness, but the examining neurologist may not detect any weakness. What is going on? If the neurologist watches the person walk, the patient may be seen dragging one leg; if the patient walks up and down the hallway without stopping, he or

Cerebellum

The part of the brain that controls movement, and enables coordinated movement. It is located behind the brain stem and under the cerebral hemispheres; it resembles a pair of tennis balls stuck to the brain stem.

The most common complaint associated with difficulty in walking is "weakness."

she may not be able to walk 100 yards. A single evaluation of a muscle may not reveal any weakness, whereas
repeated examinations may reveal prominent weakness
in the leg muscles selected for testing. This type of
assessment can be very helpful in justifying applications
for disability coverage.

If different nerve fibers are affected, such as those sensory fibers that send messages to the brain telling it
where the legs are, then the person will not be able to
control the legs. Movement might occur, but it may be
clumsy and poorly controlled and, therefore, not be
useful. This is a major problem! The patient's legs may
or may not feel "numb."

Another problem that contributes to walking difficulty,
especially early in the illness, is a lack of coordination
because of a plaque in the cerebellum (that part of the
brain just above the spinal cord inside the skull). (The
cerebellum looks like a couple of tennis balls stuck
together on top of something that looks like a fatter
spinal cord.) A plaque in the spinal cord can also cut off
fibers connecting the cerebellum to neurons in the spinal
cord, resulting in gait problems. Contrary to the common
perception, the patient does not have to have a tremor to
have difficulty walking due to a plaque in the cerebellum
or its connections.

In summary, MS plaques can affect several different
parts of the brain and spinal cord and cause difficulty
in walking.

Symptoms of Multiple Sclerosis

PART THREE

Diagnosis, Identification, and Prognosis of Multiple Sclerosis

How is a diagnosis of MS made?

What kinds of MS exist?

Do all people with MS become disabled?

More...

23. How is a diagnosis of MS made?

A diagnosis of MS is not generally accepted unless a neurologist confirms the diagnosis.

A diagnosis of MS is not generally accepted unless a neurologist confirms the diagnosis. In actuality, many general physicians are aware of the illness and recognize the characteristic problems that patients have with MS. Some have a heightened awareness of the disease, whereas others are more proficient in carrying out a neurologic exam. Nevertheless, other than neurologists with subspecialty training in MS, few have the training and experience to carry out a quantitative neurologic examination.

Regardless of who the examining physician is, certain diagnostic criteria for MS must be met to confirm the presence of this disease. The first formal criteria for the diagnosis of MS were outlined in the "Schumacher criteria." Dr. George Schumacher was the head of a National Institutes of Health (NIH) committee that was charged with coming up with simple standardized minimal criteria to be used in making a diagnosis of MS in patients entering clinical trials for MS-related therapies. The Schumacher criteria reiterated the need to establish that the lesions (plaques) were "disseminated in both time and space." In other words, to make a diagnosis of MS, there must be evidence of at least two separate affected areas in the brain and spinal cord, and the lesions must have occurred at least at two different times separated by at least 1 month. Bearing in mind that the development of these criteria preceded diagnostic imaging, satisfying them was a challenge. The primary motivation behind establishing the Schumacher criteria was to more consistently identify subjects for studies. Subsequent to their publication, these criteria were used primarily in research settings.

A little more than 20 years ago, another NIH committee focusing on MS diagnostic criteria was brought together under the chairmanship of Dr. Charles Poser. The Poser committee recognized that laboratory support for the diagnosis of MS from diagnostic imaging and improvements in spinal fluid examination represented a major advance. The terms "clinically definite," "clinically probable," and "laboratory-supported" diagnosis came into use in academic circles as a result of this understanding, though they were rarely used elsewhere.

The committee recommendations (the Poser criteria) focused interest on using magnetic resonance imaging (MRI) as well as spinal fluid **immunoglobulin** abnormalities in the diagnosis of MS. Spinal fluid analysis, however, has suffered from a lack of standardization of diagnostic testing. The Food and Drug Administration (FDA) has now outlined certain methods that must be used for detection of **oligoclonal bands** to meet the Poser criteria. These bands appear in the gamma globulin region of spinal fluid during electrophoresis testing in the laboratory. If present, they provide strong support for the diagnosis of MS. This evidence is required to confirm an MS diagnosis because proper testing is more expensive and the mandate for this testing is needed to ensure appropriate insurance coverage. Other issues related to spinal fluid testing remain to be addressed, however.

Immunoglobulin
Another word for antibody.

Oligoclonal band
Bands of antibody that are present on electrophoresis of cerebrospinal fluid.

The criteria established by the Poser committee were formulated primarily for selecting research subjects for prospective studies. An increasing number of neurologists trained in the subspecialty and their coworkers welcomed the codification of these new criteria. As a result of the revised criteria, larger numbers of patients were established as having MS.

Karen's comment:

On December 12, 1996, I began the day as a mostly healthy professor of legal ethics with a nagging case of an "inner ear virus."

31

I ended the day as an MS patient.

In between the start and the end of the day, I drove to the university to pick up my students' exams for grading and then to the doctor for him to examine my ears and give me my annual Pap test.

During that fall term, I was flying each week between New Jersey, where my husband was studying at the Princeton Theological Seminary, and Florida, where my middle sister, niece, father, and stepmother live. I taught legal ethics at New York University School of Law in the north and University of Miami School of Law in the south. For 3 months, I had extreme vertigo that was seemingly caused by "an inner ear virus." I reassured myself that when I stopped this crazy schedule, I would heal.

By December, I was taking large amounts of Antivert, Dramamine, and ginger ale to get through a 3-hour class. If I moved too fast or a student waved a hand or turned a page of a book without warning, I would fight the nausea that comes from vertigo. I memorized my lectures so that I did not have to look down at my notes. I would sometimes have to vomit during the breaks in class, wash my face, and then continue to teach.

*On the day I picked up the students' exams to grade, I went to see my general doctor. He immediately said that I did not have a **virus** and refused to let me drive myself to the emergency appointment he made with a neurologist.*

My father took me to the neurologist, who said I had either a large brain tumor or MS, and who scheduled an MRI for that day as well as a spinal tap for the next day. The MRI center was having a holiday party, and while we waited for the results to take back to the neurologist, the office

Virus

A pathogen composed of a nucleic acid genome enclosed in a protein coat. Viruses can replicate only in living cells.

administrator offered us Santa party hats and snacks to keep us distracted. My husband, who was in New Jersey, kept saying, "I thought you were having a Pap test and had a problem with your ears. What are you doing at the neurologist?" We were all a bit in shock as the surreal nature of the day continued. With MRI results and party favors in hand, we went back to the neurologist, who had waited after-hours for our return. He looked at the MRI and said, "You have MS."

The doctor asked whether I had ever had any prior events of weakness or numbness. By the time we went through his questions and my answers, a pattern of unexplained, often ignored, yet classic MS symptoms was evident. Previously, when a medical problem would get too bothersome, I would finally make an appointment with a doctor. Inevitably, the symptom went away; I was too busy to keep the appointment before it went away or an explanation emerged, and thus I canceled the appointment. I was a typical overachiever: working, making Christmas decorations by hand, entertaining my husband's corporate clients, starting a soup kitchen at our church, and keeping in touch with family each day. Fatigue was apparently due to hard work at law school and around-the-clock hours as a hostile takeover lawyer in the 1980s. Weakness in my right hand was explained as a side effect from writing a law review article and having a lumpectomy. Changes in my vision were thought to be due to long hours and the water in London causing an occasional film on my contact lenses. The inability to walk on my right foot was apparently from falling off a curb, causing a sprain that lasted 6 months. Other injuries seemingly resulted from general clumsiness, a lack of good depth perception, and so on.

Looking back, given the then-available therapies, I am not sure whether it would have mattered if I had been diagnosed earlier. Over the 20 years before my diagnosis (when I had what I now know were MS symptoms), I had completed college in 3 years, married, graduated from law school, practiced and taught law, lived overseas for 10 years, and planned a family; I had lived a "normal" life. In 1996, after 3 months of severe symptoms and with an MRI showing areas of my brain scarred from prior attacks, MS could no longer be ignored and now loomed large.

24. What is a "clinically isolated syndrome?"

Neurologists have long recognized optic neuritis (or retrobulbar neuritis) to be a forerunner of MS in the majority of such cases. Recognizing this, plus the fact that other problems such as **transverse myelitis** and acute symptoms of brain stem origin usually end up diagnosed as MS, the McDonald committee (another NIH group) has modified the Poser criteria to establish the "McDonald criteria."

The McDonald criteria embrace the rational use of laboratory investigation in making the diagnosis of MS but have abandoned the terms "clinically probable" and "laboratory-supported." The NIH committee has simply and clearly outlined MRI criteria that can be used together with a history of a single clinical attack of neurological disease (called a **clinically isolated syndrome [CIS]**) to make a diagnosis of MS with a high degree of certainty (87%). Approximately one in seven persons diagnosed with MS based on MRI criteria will not have MS, however. In all probability, most members of this small group will have experienced an attack of **acute disseminated encephalomyelitis** (a one-time "MS" attack). Recent evidence indicates that this kind of attack seems to be related to a different kind of immune reaction. We anticipate that new tests in the foreseeable future may help to distinguish individuals with acute

Transverse myelitis

Signs of spinal cord damage appearing acutely or subacutely with signs of inflammation. When accompanied by certain brain MRI abnormalities, it may qualify for a diagnosis of clinically isolated syndrome (CIS) and MS.

Clinically isolated syndrome (CIS)

Optic neuritis, acute vertigo or other isolated brain stem symptoms, or transverse myelitis. These symptoms may be considered diagnostic for MS when certain MRI abnormalities are present.

Acute disseminated encephalomyelitis

An acute spontaneous, postinfectious, or postvaccinial central nervous system disease. It is characterized by the simultaneous appearance of nervous system symptoms due to inflammation in the white matter of the brain or the spinal cord, resembling an attack of MS.

disseminated encephalomyelitis from those with true MS at the onset of illness. For example, the presence of certain cells in the spinal fluid or the presence of antibody may possibly identify such patients with even greater certainty—that is, conclusively identify those persons with illness who will not **relapse** in the future.

The decision of the committee to include MRI criteria for a CIS and to equate CIS with a diagnosis of MS was, in part, driven by the evidence from two separate studies. These are the CHAMPS study (Controlled High-Risk Avonex Multiple Sclerosis Prevention Study) of Avonex and the ETOMS (Early Treatment of Multiple Sclerosis) study of Rebif. These studies showed superior results when interferon-beta-1a treatment was started after the very first clinical attack of MS. The very low dose of Rebif in the ETOMS study yielded inferior results as compared with those found in the CHAMPS study.

The FDA has accepted initiation of treatment based on the McDonald criteria, including treatment of individuals who fall into the CIS category. The evolution and acceptance of these criteria has an important practical impact. Using the CIS criteria for diagnosis means a more favorable outcome for patients because of the better response to treatment, with its institution at the very outset of MS.

25. What are the actual new "McDonald diagnostic criteria" that neurologists use to make a diagnosis of MS?

The McDonald committee outlined the criteria in an article titled "Recommended Diagnostic Criteria," which was published in the *Annals of Neurology* journal. These

Relapse

Appearance of new signs or recurrence of previous signs of MS.

Diagnosis, Identification, and Prognosis of Multiple Sclerosis

Table 1   New MS Diagnostic Criteria

Clinical Attacks	Objective Lesions	Additional Requirements to Make Diagnosis
≥2	≥2	Clinical evidence is enough
≥2	1	Disseminated in space by MRI or + CSF and two or more MRI lesions consistent with MS or additional clinical attack in different site
1	2 or more	Disseminated in time by MRI or second clinical attack
1 Mono-symptomatic	1	Disseminated in space by MRI or + CSF and two or more MRI lesions consistent with MS and disseminated in time by MRI or second attack
0 Progressive from start	1	+ CSF and disseminated in space by MRI evidence of three or more T2 brain lesions or two or more cord lesions or four to eight brain and one cord lesions or + VEP and four to eight MS lesions or + VEP and four brain lesions + one cord lesion and disseminated in time by MRI or continued progression for 1 year

criteria have been adopted in the United States and internationally and can be obtained from the MS Society Web site. The summary of these criteria prepared by the National Multiple Sclerosis Society appears in **Table 1**.

TYPES OF MULTIPLE SCLEROSIS

26. What kinds of MS exist?

To most physicians dealing with MS and many patients, this illness seems to be a family of closely related disorders. To begin with, a doctor's clinical diagnosis of MS is based on the recognition of symptoms that recur (relapse). The relapsing nature of the disease is unique to MS. Recognition of symptoms that are typically associated with MS makes a neurologist's diagnosis easier. However, because initiation of treatment at the earliest possible time results in better outcomes, establishing the diagnosis with the first appearance of illness (CIS) is very important.

By consensus, MS is usually divided into four different types for the purposes of study: (1) relapsing–remitting MS, (2) secondary progressive MS, (3) primary progressive MS, and (4) relapsing–progressive MS. This classification system does not mean that the various types have different causes. Moreover, there are subtypes of illness within each category that may be distinguished from another based on immunological criteria or perhaps **genetic** findings.

27. If I have relapsing–remitting MS, can I get progressive disease?

Patients with relapsing–remitting illness have attacks of one or more symptoms with varying frequency and with variable degrees of recovery but, by definition, their disease does not progress between attacks. Individuals with relapsing–remitting MS have attacks without interval progression, which is the essential feature of this type of MS. If there is sustained progression between attacks, this form is considered to be secondary progressive MS. Some patients with secondary progressive disease continue to relapse.

In contrast, primary progressive MS is a type of MS in which patients have no attacks but have continually worsening disease. In this form of illness, worsening is not followed by subsequent improvement. If individuals with primary progressive disease have a subsequent attack with any recovery, they are reclassified as having

Genetic

Any issue or consideration having to do with heredity, genes, or gene changes (mutations). Also, an inherited characteristic or change.

Individuals with relapsing–remitting MS have attacks without interval progression.

Rapidly progressive MS

Also known as Marburg's variant of multiple sclerosis; a very aggressive form of MS in which the disease advances quickly and relentlessly, leading to rapid disability and death. It is also known as acute or fulminant MS.

Malignant MS

A type of MS characterized by frequent, severe relapses with a rapid increase in disability. It constitutes a very small, but important subgroup of MS.

Gene

The smallest amount of DNA in chromosomes or mitochondria that codes for a heritable characteristic or feature.

Chromosome

Structures located within the nucleus of each cell that hold genetic material.

Immunosuppressive therapy

Any treatment that results in decreased immune responses.

relapsing–progressive MS. In the future, these kinds of patients might be segregated for study as representing another category of MS. Perhaps future genetic studies may better define distinct "phenotypes" associated with specific "genotypes," but that time has not yet arrived.

It is clear that MS patients can suffer disability yet not have secondary progressive disease, as is seen in relapsing–progressive or primary progressive MS. No satisfactory terms or descriptors for stepwise progressing MS are in common use.

Rapidly progressive MS and **malignant MS** are terms that are used to describe a small minority of patients who become disabled in a short period of time. These patients typically will have three or more attacks—often severe—in their first year, and possess **gene** combinations (HLA-B-7 and DR-2) that occur in a small minority of MS patients. (They probably have inherited a whole string of MS-related genes between these chromosomal locations on **chromosome** 6.) It is particularly important that such patients be provided with expert care in MS clinics because early institution of aggressive therapy is the only way to stop the rapid progression and avoid severe permanent disability. Aggressive **immunosuppressive therapy** (**chemotherapy**) with Cytoxan (cyclophosphamide) or Novantrone (mitoxantrone) will usually stabilize them. Despite the presence of severe disability when first seen, more than one-fourth or more of these patients can experience remarkable improvement with aggressive management. **Human immunodeficiency virus (HIV)** screening is also important, as rarely patients with AIDS may have symptoms that mimic those associated with rapidly progressive MS. These individuals do not benefit from the types of treatment that can help MS patients.

28. What is chronic progressive MS?

Both secondary progressive and relapsing–progressive MS were referred to as chronic progressive disease in the past. The term "chronic progressive" is no longer used in medical circles, however. Primary progressive disease was also sometimes referred to as chronic progressive disease. Importantly, if an MS patient has never had an attack followed by a remission, he or she is diagnosed as having primary progressive MS. In contrast, if an MS patient begins with primary progressive disease, but then has an onset of new problems followed by improvement, he or she is no longer considered to have primary progression disease but rather is rediagnosed with relapsing–progressive MS.

Many neurologists in the past have concluded that there are many more types of MS, but those variations are not easily characterized or recognized clinically. Perhaps incorrectly, it has been concluded that attempting to define such subtypes will be of no help in determining prognosis or in evaluating the effects of therapy.

29. What is spinal MS?

Spinal MS was a term that was used for primary progressive MS in the past, but has not generally been used for the last 30 years or so. It was a good descriptor for this illness because the predominant symptoms are those of slowly progressive weakness and sensory problems, predominantly affecting the legs. In the past, it was especially difficult to distinguish MS from **cervical spondylosis**. Modern imaging has made this distinction much easier. For the sake of clarity, the term "primary progressive MS" is preferable because the majority of persons with this type of disease do have MRI brain lesions.

Chemotherapy
Treatment with chemicals, such as those that are used for cancer. Examples include cyclophosphamide (Cytoxan) and 6-mercaptopurine.

Human immunodeficiency virus (HIV)
The virus that causes AIDS.

Cervical spondylosis
A disease in which the disks between the vertebral bodies in the neck extrude like mortar between bricks. Sometimes the disks will compress the spinal cord, producing "MS-like" symptoms of weakness and loss of sensation in the legs. The disease process can result in pressure on nerve roots as they leave the spinal canal, resulting in weakness and/or pain in the arms and hands.

30. Who gets progressive disease without attacks?

At first, my response to this question was to assume that the person who asked this question was simply asking about the definition of this type of illness. However, he was actually asking about differences in populations and their risks of developing this type of illness. In this regard, ethnic differences are important. In France, Charcot first described the spinal form (primary progressive MS) as an "incomplete form" of MS, occurring in approximately 10% of patients. Subsequently, this form of illness was recognized as occurring in about 30% of Irish patients, and later still as occurring in about 30% of European Jews living in Israel. Primary progressive illness also appears to be more common in Spain and in persons of Spanish descent, including Cubans, who live in the United States.

Several other disorders must be distinguished from primary progressive MS. The most common of these is cervical spondylosis (compression of the spinal cord because of disc disease). Although people fear spinal cord tumors, only a tiny percentage (approximately 1%) of patients will be diagnosed as having a spinal cord tumor. Sometimes academicians introduce discussions of rare genetic disorders termed "familial spastic paraparesis" that appears as progressive disorders in childhood. Because these conditions are familial and almost always appear very early in life, they pose little difficulty for physicians who seek to distinguish them from MS. To date, more than a dozen of these disorders have been genetically and biochemically identified.

31. How will I know whether I will get progressive disease?

The absence of attacks with new neurologic symptoms, or recurrence of older problems, does not necessarily mean that a person has progressive MS. Patients with disability can be stable for long periods of time. To recognize progression in MS, neurologic difficulties must be worsening. To determine whether a patient has progressed or changed neurologically, a neurologist must perform sequential examinations of the patient over a period of several months. The patient must undergo a complete quantitative neurologic examination to deter-mine and then record disability scores, which are then compared with scores from previous and future exam-inations. It takes special training to perform such examinations with consistency and to provide usable information. The patient with progressive disease can assist in this process by pointing out to the neurologist which types of problems are progressing. However, if the ability to walk distances is becoming increasingly limited, in the absence of another explanation, pro-gression of MS is likely.

To recognize progression in MS, neurologic difficulties must be worsening.

Why patients with primary progressive disease do not ordinarily experience attacks is unknown. Actually, roughly one-third of the patients who originally experi-ence only progressive problems subsequently do experi-ence one or more exacerbations, but when they do, they have relatively few. It is possible that those persons who never have acute attacks have a different type of disease process that involves antibody-mediated **demyelination** independent of lymphocytes. At the present, this con-jecture is purely speculative.

Demyelination

The loss of myelin surrounding the axon, or nerve fiber, regardless of the disease process.

In addition to those patients with primary progressive MS, many patients with secondary progressive illness stop having clear-cut attacks and notice that their disease begins to progress, often in a waxing-and-waning fashion. After a dozen years of illness, progression and attacks may no longer be evident to either the patient or the physician. Evidence of progression by examination may be difficult to detect in many patients. Longer-term observation of these patients may reveal continued worsening; that is, neurologic functions that appear to be preserved may actually be partially lost.

PROGNOSIS AND DISABILITY

32. Do all people with MS become disabled?

Some neurologists, many in academic circles, have a perception that MS is predictably associated with disability. Before the advent of new testing procedures, particularly MRI of the brain and spinal cord, many patients were not diagnosed with this disease during their lifetimes. Without proven treatments, outside of academic centers there was little incentive to make such a diagnosis in those persons without disability. The training of many more neurologists in recent years has led to greater availability of neurologic consultation; therefore, a larger proportion of previously undiagnosed patients are now correctly recognized as having MS. Thus, in the past, those persons who had more evidence of disability than the majority were correctly diagnosed; those who were minimally affected were not. Now that a variety of treatments are available, the importance of early diagnosis and treatment is widely accepted, and a larger number of patients are being correctly diagnosed as having MS.

In my experience, general physicians previously gave approximately two-thirds of the women who were diagnosed with MS an initial "psychiatric" label. Now, with the advantages of increasing numbers of physicians (neurologists) trained to recognize MS and the general availability of MRI equipment, many more people are recognized as having this disorder. In Europe, where large numbers of patients have been cared for in specialty centers, it is now evident that the majority of these people with MS are not disabled. The inclusion of patients with milder illness that might not have been diagnosed previously as part of the "MS population" is a factor contributing to lower levels of disability in patients and better outcomes in more recent studies with placebo therapies as well as with active treatment.

Karen's comment:

I hate to think of myself as disabled, but I am. The tests for disability and levels of disability include the EDSS scale, the U.S. government Social Security definitions, societal measures, and our own internal meters. Each has biases, limits, and uses. Due to an unusual set of circumstances, I do not qualify for U.S. Social Security but do have entitlement to some U.K. "incapacity benefit." The way this is measured includes how well and how long I am able to pour hot water from a "kettle"; that is, if I cannot make a proper cup of tea, I am considered incapacitated!

I was at a talk where Dr. Crayton asked how many people there used or had disability stickers. I viewed myself proudly as someone who had one but did not use it. Dr. Crayton told my category to "get over yourself" and noted that even if you save yourself one step, using the sticker could translate into a better quality of life. I have also had people glare at me when we use the sticker and they can't tell how hard it is for me to function.

At my worst, I have been a 5.5 on the EDSS, and at my best, a 1.5. Sometimes I think I have "aced" the testing

Dr. Sheremata gives me, only to have him ask about things he has noticed. I wish I could always pass the tests with a 1, make a perfect cup of tea, and not be bothered by what others think a disability sticker means or how I label myself. I try to keep in mind that the goal, unlike other tests, is not to pass; it is to learn—to find out how I am, and deal with it.

In 2006, in connection with the FDA hearings about returning Tysabri to the market, several national news teams came to our home to film my husband and me. They wanted to show, among other things, what "disabled" meant. When they arrived, I was dressed and barefoot, and lying down until the filming began. The camera crew felt it would help to show, as an outtake, my husband helping me get ready; because the programs were G-rated, that meant putting on my shoes. We told the camera crew I usually go barefoot to help me walk and feel the ground, even in the New England weather, but they felt our sense of doing things as a couple and the struggles to function at times could be portrayed in this way. The somewhat hardened crew teared up as David helped me sit up. They smiled when they began to get an idea of his "fraternity guy" approach to caretaking when he wiped my face with a corner of his sleeve. As he tried to put my feet into "peds," which shot across the room like rubber bands at each of his attempts, they laughed aloud. We did the filming with me barefoot, disabled, but—we were told by the television producers—still able to communicate.

33. How long will it be before I will be disabled?

Recently, there has been speculation that disability in MS patients will be predictably present after several years of illness. Some have claimed that there is no difference between various patient groups and that disability eventually occurs in the majority of patients.

Apart from this rhetoric, it is clear that the rate of progression in the early years of the illness is in part related to the number of relapses during the beginning of the illness. The Canadian observation that a single relapse in the first year of illness is a good prognostic sign is one that the majority of neurologists who are experienced in the care of MS share. In the "population studies" in southern Ontario, three attacks in the first year of illness led to wheelchair dependence within 5 years in half of those patients. This finding is in agreement with the clinical observation that an unusually large number of MS attacks in a short time period predict unusually severe disease.

Genetic studies have shown that patients with aggressive MS are genetically distinguished by the presence of two genes together: HLA-B7 and DR-2 (DR-1 1501). Both of these genes are located on the short arm of chromosome 6 close to each other, indicating that a large number of genes related to immune function and located in this region are probably inherited together: the so-called linkage disequilibrium. The study of genes in this region relative to the various MS subtypes should be highly productive.

Recent studies of large numbers of patients in Europe, who were followed and documented for decades, have produced "new" data. These data from Europe indicate that 30% of patients will develop progressive disease, rather than a larger percentage estimated by centers in the United States. It is important to bear in mind that these observations are based primarily on "untreated" MS patients. In other words, these patients have not benefited from taking drugs that have been proven to reduce attacks of MS and to reduce the risk of disability.

Large numbers of neurologists interested in MS in the United States, Canada, and Europe have come to the same conclusions regarding the prognosis of MS:

- Women with MS do better than men!
- The onset of MS before the age of 30 is associated with a better prognosis.
- Having just one attack of MS in the first year of illness predicts less disability.
- Optic neuritis or retrobulbar neuritis as an initial attack is associated with a good prognosis.
- A low lesion load (numbers of lesions and/or lesion volume) identified by MRI is associated with a better outlook.

34. Why do some people get worse so quickly? Will I?

There are probably many reasons why the condition of some people with MS worsens more quickly than the condition of others. Apart from those persons who are genetically predisposed to progress rapidly, stress is an important factor. Stress has been implicated in many other diseases, and without question, it plays an important role in MS.

It is clear that some patients are genetically predisposed to rapid progression of illness. Persons who have the DR-2 (DR-1 1501) gene have more severe disease than those who do not. Almost 40 years ago, Dr. Dupont (in Denmark) showed that when MS patients have both the DR-2 and HLA-B7 genes, they predictably have rapidly progressive disease and severe disability (malignant MS). For example, in our Florida experience, although only 7% of Cuban patients in our study sample had the DR-2 gene, when they had both the DR-2 and HLB-B7 genes, these patients developed malignant MS.

There is no simple way of determining beforehand how an individual patient will fare during the course of MS. The frequency of attacks (one attack in the first year), good recovery from the attack, a small amount of disease in brain MRI scans, and recovery of a feeling of well-being are good indicators for a better outlook. The longer the remission, the greater the likelihood of a sustained remission. Treatment has improved the outlook for all MS patients. This is especially true for those with the worst forms of disease!

There is no simple way of determining beforehand how an individual patient will fare during the course of MS.

35. Is memory affected with MS?

Memory can be affected by MS. Confusion can accompany attacks and can be associated with memory difficulty, but this effect is not defined as true memory impairment. Rather, it is associated with generally impaired **cognition**. Anxiety and depression also can rob a person of his or her ability to maintain attention. When the anxiety or depression abates, memory returns to normal. Even so, memory complaints tend to increase with the duration of MS and its accompanying disability.

Cognition
The ability to reason.

The Avonex CHAMPS trial was the first to document that early treatment in the course of the illness can prevent cognitive impairment. In that trial, patients were treated if they had an optic neuritis and two or more plaques seen in an MRI (i.e., at the very onset of their illness). No cognitive difficulty was seen in patients prior to treatment, but placebo-treated patients, as a group, had detectable cognitive difficulty after 1 year.

Karen's comment:

I used to be smart. When I try to barter with God about my MS, I offer walking in exchange for my memory. When I get sad, angry, depressed, or frustrated with MS, it is usually about my cognitives. When I want my pre-MS self back, it is my intelligence I long for.

In 1996, when I was first diagnosed, I had trouble reading—not surprising given the vertigo, limited vision, and medications. After these symptoms subsided, I still had trouble reading—not problems seeing the words, but rather processing the words. By the time I would finish a page, I had no idea what I had read. Cognitive problems were not mentioned or referred to in anything I researched about MS. Dr. Sheremata validated my experience and suggested neuropsychiatric testing to ascertain my cognitive status.

The test results revealed that my long-term memory and even short-term memory were fine, but my short-term working memory was a problem. It was reassuring to know that I was not imagining this, but it was shocking to see the numbers in print—my short-term working memory was in the bottom 16%! What this translates into is difficulty learning new information (phone numbers, names, and places where my things are moved), processing new information (understanding a new or unanticipated item), manipulating information (changing times for an event), making decisions (determining what to have for dinner), and transferring data (addressing an envelope). I can use some other parts of my brain to compensate or almost mask what is occurring, but if I am physically tired or challenged, I do not have cells available, and my cognitive functioning "floods." Moreover, it is not easy to explain to others that my cognitives are shutting down.

In the last few years, cognitive problems with MS have become more widely recognized. However, this topic is still not easily discussed; cognition goes to the core of who we are, and often people do not want to acknowledge or even know about it. I have been at MS support group meetings where bladder control and **erectile dysfunction** are discussed openly and with ease. If I mention cognition, the room goes silent, and no one wants to talk about it.

In addition to acknowledging cognitive loss, I manage this MS symptom with medication, compensatory techniques, and rehabilitation. The medications I tried for cognition had not been studied for MS at the time I took them. However, with my doctor's supervision, I took Aricept and memantine. These and other medications currently are being investigated for use with MS.

As for compensatory techniques, the expert advice is not very advanced. The best suggestion that they offer is to keep a "to do" list, something a lifelong obsessive–compulsively organized person like me has been doing forever! I also have routines and systems to remind me to take medicines, that I have an appliance working, and how to reorient myself when I get on cognitive overload.

I tried structured cognitive rehabilitation—even going to an Alzheimer's disease clinic—for many months to see whether their techniques could have application to my MS, but unfortunately this did not help. Additionally, I have used different programs for "brain training," including ones available at no charge through Web sites such as myMSmyWay, Lumosity, and PositScience.

The best practical help I have gotten for cognition came when I met with a psychologist (with the incongruous name of Dr. Payne), who helped me develop rehabilitation techniques. We took certain activities (most of which I was unfamiliar with) and combined them, trying to create new pathways in my brain, retrain and reinforce old pathways, and establish new skills to have as backups to existing pathways. For example, I memorize verses; take piano lessons;

Erectile dysfunction

The repeated inability to get or keep an erection firm enough to complete sexual intercourse. The word "impotence" is used to describe other problems that interfere with sexual intercourse and reproduction, such as lack of sexual desire and problems with ejaculation or orgasm. Using the term "erectile dysfunction" makes it clear that those other problems are not involved.

do origami, needlepoint, and jigsaw puzzles; play card games; and juggle. As I improve in these functions, I try to do these tasks and add in a second or third cognitive process such as listening to NPR or a recorded book in the background. It is humbling to struggle through things many kindergartners do with ease. It is both frustrating and a bit frightening when I find myself unable to recall how to do the task or to start to "melt down" as I re-re-re-remember the song I played last month on the piano. However, it can also be empowering to finally be able to master turning a piece of paper into a bunny or a series of notes on a page into music.

Recently, my husband came home and said, "What a great origami bird. I think you've got it. I am so proud." At first, I shared in this feeling of triumph. Then reality hit, and I gave him a twofold response: "(A) this is not a bird: it is a flower, and (B) I did not go to law school for 3 years to make paper toys!" Before MS, I was smart with little effort; now it is enough to try to be smart about the loss of my cognitive ability and to do what I can to retain and retrain it.

36. How long will I be able to walk? Will I become paralyzed and end up in a wheelchair?

The ability to walk is affected in an increasing proportion of untreated MS patients over time, but the rate of progression varies from patient to patient. Frequent attacks with incomplete recovery are indicators of a poorer outlook. Importantly, the likelihood of disability is diminished by (early) therapeutic intervention.

The studies of the natural history of MS in patients in southern Ontario documented that half of those who had three attacks within their first year required the use of wheelchairs within 5 years of onset. In reality, those (untreated) patients will often be wheelchair bound within 2 years. This kind of progression warrants an aggressive approach to MS management. These patients should be *referred early* to MS centers, which are experienced in the use of aggressive measures to treat this disease. Aggressive use of immunosuppression can be remarkably effective in stopping progression. However, if the patient has already developed fixed severe disability, stabilization will have less meaning. At that point, the appropriate goals may have already become impossible to achieve. One-fourth to one-third of patients will exhibit functional improvement if such treatment is initiated within a few months of onset of malignant MS. Knowledge of specific complications, taking steps to avoid them, and the appropriate follow-up are essential for the safe implementation of such aggressive measures. The newest drug for MS, Tysabri (natalizumab), has been used for maintenance of immunosuppression after induction with Cytoxan or Novantrone. Results appear favorable.

37. Will I regain my bladder control?

The loss of bladder function occurs in a proportion of patients with MS. With acute attacks where control of voiding is lost, recovery often follows promptly. However, from several older studies of (untreated) patients with long-term follow-up, it is apparent that eventually two-thirds of all MS patients may be left with some impairment of bladder function.

Expert care of the bladder is important in all patients. Prompt and effective management of infections and measures taken to prevent infections are primary goals. Many urologists are less interested in medical **urology** and often lack appropriate diagnostic equipment to

Urology

The field of medical care dealing with diseases of the kidneys, bladder, and associated structures including the ureters and urethra. In men, this field also deals with diseases of the male reproductive organs.

evaluate patients fully. Urinary frequency may not indicate the presence of infection, and the use of antibiotics without verifying the presence of infection will contribute to the development of resistant organisms. All patients with bladder or kidney infections should have appropriate urine specimens submitted for examination and culture before taking antibiotics. If the organism identified appears to be resistant to the antibiotic originally prescribed and the patient is not responding to treatment, a more appropriate antibiotic can be selected based on the culture report. Upon completion of antibiotic treatment follow-up cultures are important to ensure that the infection is resolved. With effective treatment of infection, the bladder is likely to function more normally than one that is chronically irritated. Drugs that reduce the irritability of the bladder can be helpful but do not replace antibiotics as treatment for infections.

The use of antibiotics related to Cipro and Levaquin (the fluoroquinolone antibiotics, which now number more than three dozen on the market) is unwise. Dr. Barry Arnason, of the University of Chicago, recognized the greater frequency of MS relapses when these antibiotics were used. In my practice, we have also documented a high frequency of severe relapses following the use of these antibiotics. The fluoroquinolone antibiotics induce increased production of interferon-gamma—and a prospective trial of interferon-gamma conducted by University of Maryland researchers resulted in increased frequency of relapse. Thus it is clear that this group of antibiotics should not be used in MS patients, except in life-saving situations where resistance to other organisms is reported.

PART FOUR

Causes of Multiple Sclerosis

Do viruses cause MS?

What is the role of the immune system in MS?

Is MS hereditary?

More . . .

Epstein-Barr virus (EBV)

A member of the herpesvirus family that is one of the most common viruses infecting humans. The virus occurs worldwide, and most people become infected with it sometime during their lives.

Environmental factor

Any factor in the environment that may contribute to the risk of a disease, such as MS. The environmental factor in MS is assumed to be a virus.

Hereditary

Transmitted from parent to child by information contained in the genes. See *gene* and *genetics*.

38. What causes MS?

Since the publication of the first edition of this book, considerable strides have been made in understanding the genetic basis of the predisposition to MS. There have also been substantial advances in immunology, particularly in relationship to control or regulation of immune responses. Although there has been renewed interest in immune responses to the **Epstein-Barr virus (EBV)**, there has been no strong evidence implicating this virus, either directly or indirectly, as a cause of MS.

There are no simple answers to the questions "What causes MS?" and "Why do some people get MS?" Over the last century and a half, three important interrelated contributing factors have been recognized: **environmental factors** (usually thought to be infectious), immune factors, and **hereditary** (genetic) factors. Obviously, it would be impossible to do more than superficially discuss these issues given the limited amount of space available here. Instead, just the most commonly asked questions are addressed.

Population studies have yielded information from which it has been inferred that an environmental factor exists. Persons moving from high-risk to low-risk areas take the risk with them if they move after the age of 15 years. Conversely, if they move before the age of 15 years, they appear to leave the risk behind. This information comes from studies of populations moving from Europe (a high-risk area) to Africa (a low-risk area). Similar observations have been noted in populations moving into Israel. These findings, as well as the occurrence of an epidemic of MS in the Faroe Islands after the "invasion" of those islands by British troops at the outset of World War II, suggest that an infectious agent plays a role in MS.

INFECTIONS AND MULTIPLE SCLEROSIS

39. Do viruses cause MS?

The onset of an acute demyelinating disease (post-infectious **encephalomyelitis**) occurs after a number of different infections, such as measles and mumps as well as smallpox **vaccination**. Approximately one-fourth of all persons who are diagnosed with **postinfectious encephalomyelitis** eventually wind up with a diagnosis of MS. This link has naturally raised suspicions that viruses might be the cause of MS. Over the years, research has implicated many infectious agents, such as the measles virus (and other paramyxoviruses), **distemper**, the T-cell leukemia virus, and certain **bacteria**, as possible environmental factors. For the most part, these candidates have been discarded. No single infection is known to cause MS. Nevertheless, there is now renewed interest in the related herpesviruses, the Epstein-Barr virus (EBV) and human herpes simplex 6 virus (HSV-6). A number of scientific papers over the last two decades, particularly in the last few years, have implicated roles for these agents in MS but have not established causation.

40. What does herpes (virus) have to do with MS?

The **herpes** families of viruses include DNA viruses that, once inside the human body, persist there for the rest of the person's life. Although herpes simplex type 1 (HSV-1) and type 2 (HSV-2) can live in neurons and seem to be protected by them, there is no evidence that they or another family of herpesviruses (**cytomegaloviruses**) have any potential role in the causation or reactivation of MS. Although another herpesvirus (the chicken pox [zoster] virus) can cause demyelination in

Encephalomyelitis
An illness associated with inflammation of the brain and spinal cord.

Vaccination
The deliberate induction of adaptive immunity to a pathogen by injecting a vaccine, a dead or attenuated (nonpathogenic) form of the pathogen.

Postinfectious encephalomyelitis
Acute disseminated encephalomyelitis occurring following an infection.

Distemper
Illness in dogs and cats caused by the measles-like distemper paramyxovirus of the same name.

Bacteria
Microscopic infectious organisms that cause a variety of diseases in humans and other species.

Herpes
Any of several species of herpesviruses (DNA viruses) that are responsible for diseases including chicken pox, shingles, mononucleosis, oral herpes (fever blisters or cold sores, HSV-1), and roseola infantum.

Causes of Multiple Sclerosis

Cytomegaloviruses

A family of herpesviruses that inhabit the urinary tract of almost all humans. Several subtypes have been described and appear to have geographic distributions.

Lymph glands

Collections of lymphocytes in organs of immune function; also called lymph nodes. They are numerous in certain parts of the body including the neck, axillae (arm pits), and groin.

Myelin basic protein

A structural protein of myelin. It is the most antigenic protein in myelin, meaning it is the most potent protein capable of stimulating the immune system. It is highly effective in minuscule amounts in producing experimental (auto)allergic encephalomyelitis, an experimental form of MS.

rare circumstances, this virus has no demonstrated role in MS. In the last few years, attention has turned to other herpesviruses—specifically, the Epstein-Barr virus (EBV) and herpes simplex virus 6 (HSV-6).

41. My doctor told me that I have antibody to the Epstein-Barr virus. Why do I have this antibody if I have MS?

All of us encounter the Epstein-Barr virus at some point in our lives. Very young children and persons past college age may not have any symptoms accompanying their infection, but adolescents and young adults characteristically experience marked fatigue and have large **lymph glands** with the infection. Antibody levels in most infected people fall and may seem to disappear over a long period of time. However, many patients with MS have higher than normal levels of this antibody (including "early" antibodies to EBV as well as to many other viruses and substances). It has been generally accepted that this antibody appears to be due to a problem of the immune responses rather than indicating that EBV is playing a role in MS. That is, the antibody is not a "neutralizing antibody" indicative of a recent or recurrent infection. Recently, some scientists have reported that one-third of MS patients have a type of virus antibody in their spinal fluid that is not present in persons without MS. The importance of this finding is uncertain.

Other exciting work has shown immunologic cross-reactivity of MS patients' lymphocytes between EBV and **myelin basic protein** (a protein found in the brain). In other words, the human immune system reacts to a protein in the EBV virus and can cross-react with a brain protein (so-called molecular mimicry), thereby producing myelin damage. No final conclusions about these findings have been reached. Two recent papers have reported that early nuclear antibody levels increase with attacks of MS and the level of this antibody, as correlated with the measured volume of active brain lesions (plaques). A very recent report stating that neutralizing antibody levels increase with attacks has not been confirmed. More investigation in this area is needed.

42. What is the importance of HSV-6 in MS?

Currently, a great deal of interest is in the newly recognized family of viruses known as herpes simplex virus 6 (HSV-6). This virus family is distantly related to HSV-1 (the cold sore virus) but is very closely related to EBV and yet another family of viruses called HSV-7. Both HSV-6 and the other closely related virus (HSV-7) share two-thirds of their DNA structure with the EBV virus. Cross-reactivity of antibody to these viruses might be one explanation of the finding of "antibody to EBV" in MS. HSV-6 and HSV-7, as well as EBV, can infect the cells of the immune system (lymphocytes) and stimulate them to uncontrolled reproduction (immortalize them). Although all three viruses can infect the immune system and immortalize lymphocytes, only HSV-6 and HSV-7 can infect cells in the nervous system. The HSV-6 virus has been found in the cells that make myelin—the oligo-dendrocytes—of MS patients. Research into a possible role for EBV, HSV-6, and other related viruses continues. No convincing relationship of HSV-6 or HSV-7 to causation of MS has, as yet, been established, but this remains an active and important area of research. Because of the genetic similarity of HSV-6, HSV-7, and EBV, investigations in this area are difficult.

HSV-6 ordinarily affects children younger than the age of 2 and is the cause of *roseola infantum*, an illness characterized by high fever and rash. Epidemiological studies have shown that HSV-7 affects children between the ages of four and six, but the virus has not been associated with illness. EBV has been extensively studied for the last three decades and plays a role in both lymphoma and infectious mononucleosis. Further study of all three viruses in MS is urgently needed.

43. Is chlamydia a cause of MS?

Chlamydia
pneumoniae

A bacterium that can cause pneumonia and that has been studied as a potential factor in MS as well as some other diseases. It is not the organism that causes genital infections in men and women.

Acinetobacter

A bacterium that infects the upper respiratory tract and that has been hypothesized to be a causative factor in MS by some researchers in England.

Chlamydia pneumoniae and, more recently, *Acinetobacter* are other organisms that have been implicated by research as playing a role in MS. The type of chlamydia (*C. pneumoniae*) that is being studied in MS is not the organism that commonly causes sexually transmitted disease (*C. trachomatis*). Although research in this area continues, these agents have not been shown to play any specific role in MS.

IMMUNITY AND MULTIPLE SCLEROSIS

44. What is the role of the immune system in MS?

A great deal of evidence has been accumulated over the last several decades indicating that abnormal immune reactions against myelin proteins can be detected in patients with MS. Although antibodies to myelin are common in patients with MS, they are also common in patients with other disorders as well.

The occurrence of inflammatory disease of the brain and spinal cord (acute encephalomyelitis) following infections and immunizations (especially after the use of a killed-virus rabies vaccine made from rabbit spinal cord) led to studies of the "allergic" potential of certain proteins in the nervous system. Most research has been focused on a single protein—myelin basic protein—because it has a high potential for the induction of experimental demyelinating disease in rats, guinea pigs, monkeys, and other animals. Only 10-millionths of a gram (there are 450 grams in 1 pound) injected into a genetically susceptible rat can result in experimental disease resembling MS. More than 30 years ago, researchers discovered that cells reactive to this protein are found in the blood of MS patients. More recently, Swedish scientists have found cells with similar reactivity in the spinal fluid of MS patients. Importantly, the original research in this area was translated into a treatment (Copaxone) that is now approved for use in MS. Copaxone is a synthetic "fake" brain protein that serves as a decoy to redirect immune reactions away from myelin basic protein in myelin.

In recent years, other nervous system proteins have been implicated in autoallergic central nervous system diseases. A large myelin protein (**proteolipid**) has been used to induce experimental disease. More than a dozen **mutations** (changes in the structure of the DNA with the potential to alter the normal function of the gene coding for this protein) have been found in different families with **familial infantile spastic paraplegia**, a nervous system disease that superficially resembles MS. Despite this advance in understanding of those rare disorders, this myelin protein does not seem to have any importance in MS. In fact, immune responses to this protein in MS patients are difficult to detect and, when they are found, do not occur more commonly in patients with MS than in patients with other nervous system diseases.

There is continuing interest focused on another protein found in miniscule quantities in the central

Causes of Multiple Sclerosis

Proteolipid
A structural protein of myelin. It can be used to sensitize mice and produce an experimental form of allergic encephalomyelitis.

Mutation
A change in the structure of DNA with a potential to alter the normal function of the gene.

Familial infantile spastic paraplegia
A group of different genetic disorders that cause spasticity in family members, usually occurring in infancy. Early onset in a family setting ordinarily easily distinguishes these rare disorders from MS.

*Autoimmunity
is an immune
reaction
against "self."*

nervous system called **myelin oligodendrocyte glyco-protein (MOG)**. Monkeys immunized with MOG protein develop a disease more closely resembling the human disease of MS than disease induced with myelin basic protein. Studies reporting the presence of antibody to this protein have not confirmed the same antibody to be present in the blood of human patients with their first manifestation of illness (MS). This is particularly disappointing because MOG antibody is capable of transferring disease in primates. Antibody to MOG is found in a high proportion of human patients with progressive MS, however. Research continues in this area, even though a firm role for anti-MOG antibody has not been established. However, there is a suspicion that immune reactions to MOG accompany immune reactions to myelin basic protein. Immune response to both proteins may be of importance in a subset of patients.

45. What is autoimmunity?

Autoimmunity is an immune reaction against "self." Autoimmune disease implies that tissue damage is a result of an autoimmune (autoallergic) reaction. This may be the result of antibody production or as a result of lymphocytes (CD4+) causing damage directly or in concert with macrophages. In a third type of immunologic reaction, known as antibody-mediated tissue damage, different lymphocytes (CD8+) cause additional damage. All three types of reactions are thought to play a role in some patients with MS. Recent evidence implicates CD8+ cells in attacks of demyelinating disease called acute disseminated encephalomyelitis. Although it resembles MS, this disease does not have a relapsing course. Instead, it is like a "single attack of an MS" type of disease.

It has also been postulated that another type of lymphocyte, known as T-helper 17 (Th17) cells, which appear to play an important role in **rheumatoid arthritis** and in **Crohn's disease**, may play an important role in MS. Convincing evidence for a role for Th17 cells and inter-leukin-17 (IL-17) in MS has not been advanced as yet. It is quite possible that the Th17 cell population and the production of the chemical messenger IL-17 may be important in a subset of patients with more aggressive disease.

Platelets may also play a role in the disease process in patients with more severe MS, as is the case in rheuma-toid arthritis and Crohn's disease.

Evidence for innate immune responses initiated within the human nervous system is well established. The role of this type of immune response in MS remains rather ill defined, however. Microglial cells in the brain, which correspond to macrophages found elsewhere in the body, can respond to interferon-gamma produced by other cells in the brain called astrocytes. Despite this potential, blocking lymphocytes from the blood-stream by Tysabri benefits MS patients—a fact that suggests the innate immune responses are of lesser importance. Nevertheless, strong evidence indicates damage caused by macrophages is a primary factor in nervous system damage. Most of these cells enter the nervous system from the blood, but some of these cells are resident in the brain and spinal cord. Currently, several studies are focused on defining the role of resi-dent macrophages in the nervous system.

46. Do antibodies cause MS?

For a long time, antibody was considered to be a likely cause of myelin damage in MS, but this theory eventu-ally fell out of favor. More recently, stronger evidence has been gathered showing that an antibody to a newly rec-ognized myelin protein (anti-MOG antibody) may play

Rheumatoid arthritis
A common inflamma-tory joint disease caused by an autoim-mune response.

Crohn's disease
An autoimmune inflammatory disease that principally, but not exclusively, affects the small bowel. It occurs with increased frequency in MS patients.

Causes of Multiple Sclerosis

a role in some patients. Additional evidence comes from analysis of brain tissue from patients in whom antibody has been deposited on myelin and an antibody-mediated, CD8+ lymphocyte type of **pathology** is present. It is not known whether this antibody is truly anti-MOG, but anti-MOG antibody was recently detected in the blood of patients at the very outset of their illness. Other studies have shown that a high proportion of patients with progressive MS also have this antibody in their blood. However, its presence does not necessarily mean that the antibody is *causing* the myelin damage.

A specific antibody (NMO-Ig) has been found in most people who have a form of severe demyelinating disease known as neuromyelitis optica (or Devic's disease). This antibody is aimed at a single-molecule water pump called aquaporin-4. Antibody to this water pump accounts for the tremendous swelling of the optic nerves and spinal cord characteristic of Devic's disease. This swelling often results in blindness or complete paralysis of the legs. In the past, Devic's disease has been thought of as a form of MS; more recently, it has been accepted as a separate entity with a specific antibody marker, unlike MS. Nevertheless, the majority of patients with Devic's disease are misdiagnosed as having MS, at least initially. Early introduction of more aggressive therapy is very effective in rolling back disability and preventing future increased disability in such cases.

47. What causes an MS plaque?

The typical MS plaque seen in patients who have died early in their illness or who have had brain biopsies is composed of a mixture of lymphocytes with many more macrophages, without antibody. The macrophages in the plaque contain myelin within their cell bodies in various stages of digestion. Some axons are damaged, but they

Pathology

The scientific study of disease. Also, detectable damage to tissues.

are relatively preserved as compared with myelin. After the initial insult by these cells, scarring begins. This process varies greatly from one individual to another. Curiously, the macrophages contain hormones, such as **brain-derived nerve growth factor (BDNGF)**, that should stimulate repair. The macrophage also secretes another hormone that stimulates scarring (**T-cell growth factor beta-1**). The invading cells seeking to remove some unknown enemy virus or protein seem prepared to help in rebuilding the damaged tissue.

Later in the development of the plaque, scarring occurs. It is this scarring that makes the plaque hard (**sclerotic**). The contraction of the scar has the potential to strangle many nerve fibers as the fibers contract over a period of many months.

In summary, the plaque is an area of intense inflammation with myelin damage, where the nerve fibers are relatively preserved and show variable amounts of scarring.

48. Is there a connection between a virus infection and autoimmune disease?

A comment about the relationship of virus infection to autoimmune disease in general is warranted. Infectious mononucleosis occurs only when adolescents or young adults are infected with EBV. The symptoms of infectious mononucleosis (and other autoimmune phenomena) occur as a result of the immune reaction to the viral infection. Dr. Gertrude Henle, who discovered the relationship between EBV and infectious mononucleosis, studied a possible link between MS and this virus; she concluded that there was no such link. Research in this area continues, however, because investigators have noted consistently high antibody titers to a specific part of EBV in many patients with MS. Very recently, a

Brain-derived nerve growth factor (BDNGF)

A specific nervous system hormone that can stimulate repair of the nervous system. It was originally found in the brain, but more recently has been found to be produced by cells causing inflammation in the brain.

T-cell growth factor beta-1

An interleukin (hormone) produced by lymphocytes that stimulates scarring in tissues. It also stimulates myelin formation.

Sclerotic

A term referring to hardened tissue, such as MS plaques in the brain. This hardness or sclerosis is caused by scarring.

correlation between levels of the antibody and the volume of active brain disease has been reported. These factors do not correlate with levels of neutralizing antibody—that is, antibody that would eliminate the virus.

EBV, HSV-6, and HSV-7 are very closely related families of viruses. Indeed, the structures of EBV, HSV-6, and HSV-7 are two-thirds identical, which has made progress in understanding the potential role of the agents difficult to achieve.

Apart from immune responses to the virus itself, an immune reaction to proteins liberated from brain tissue damaged by an immune reaction has been theorized to cause damage to myelin as well as other tissues. There is now good evidence in experimental animals and in humans that this presumption is correct.

Another theory is that part of the protein in a virus is similar in some aspect—or even identical—to a natural protein in myelin or other tissue. As noted previously, an immune reaction to two seemingly dissimilar proteins, a myelin protein and a component of EBV, has been documented. Antibody to a protein made by an EBV gene cross-reacts with part of the myelin basic protein molecule. This protein has been made synthetically and has been used to produce MS-like disease in rodents. An immune response to the virus, therefore, *can* result in myelin damage. It is possible that regulation or control of immune responses to this viral protein may be genetically impaired to a greater or lesser degree in certain patients. Obviously, further study of this issue is needed.

Researchers have theorized that a virus, from which children are protected early in life, infects adolescents who are genetically predisposed to develop MS. This virus infection results in an immune reaction to one or more proteins in the virus that resemble proteins in myelin, initiating the attack on the person's own myelin that is characteristic of MS. This immune attack then leads to additional damage to myelin (and other nervous system tissue). The damage to normal tissues is followed by additional immune reactions and more potential attacks. Immunologists think that an important part of this problem is an ineffective control of the immune reaction in MS patients, which allows additional attacks to occur.

GENETICS AND MULTIPLE SCLEROSIS

49. Is MS hereditary?

Excitement has surrounded *The International MS Genetics Consortium* large scale genome wide association scan (GWAS) studies. Using **single-nucleotide polymorphisms (SNPs**; pronounced as "snips") as "tags" for genes hypothesized to play a role in MS; this research has confirmed the association of many immune system genes with an increased risk of MS. The majority of these genes are located on the short arm of chromosome 6 at the "p21" location; classically referred to as the "Major Histocompatibility Complex (MHC) locus." Simply; these MHC gene loci are referred to as MHC class I (HLA-A, B, and C) and class II (DR) locus genes; with the class I genes appearing to be primarily concerned with antibody and class II with cellular immunity. Research has also identified important "risk" genes outside this region including the interleukin-2r, interleukin-7r, and interferon-γr receptor genes. Other newly discovered genes appear to have a protective function for MS.

Single-nucleotide polymorphism (SNP)

Any of a group of gene alterations that may be a "signature group" for a disease.

Causes of Multiple Sclerosis

Genetic factors have been recognized as playing a role in MS for many years. Although MS is typically a disease associated with European ancestry, it also occurs in African Americans; sharing genes commonly found in both African and European populations. That MS is half as common in African Americans as in white Americans correlates with a risk related to European ancestry. Among Europeans, MS is much more common in those who live in northwestern Europe, particularly in Scandinavia, Scotland, and Ireland. However, as physicians trained in neurology returned to areas in southern Europe that were initially considered to be low-risk areas, such as Sardinia and Sicily, MS became diagnosed much more often. Indeed, these two areas, as well as Madrid, Spain, are now "high-risk" areas for MS. These observations have been interpreted as evidence that both hereditary factors and environmental factors affect the risk of MS.

Certain specific genes are more common in MS patient populations. It has been known that the genes HLA-A3, HLA-B7, and DR-2 (15), which are all located on chromosome 6, are twice as common in patients with MS. They are sometimes referred to "risk factors" for MS but the majority of persons with these genes do *not* have MS. This clearly indicates there are not "MS genes." Several years ago, the DR gene was proven to be an immune response gene. DR-2 (specifically identified as DR-1*15:01) is simply a genetic mutation of the immune response gene that is twice as common in MS. The HLA-A3 gene is now known to be part of the DR1*15:01 complex. However, a number of other genes, independent of DR1*15:01 have been shown to be associated with an increased risk of MS. It has been suggested that certain mutations of immune response genes are more efficient in their function in turning on immune responses, as least as far as reactions to nervous system proteins. It has also been surmised that each gene contributes a cumulative risk for MS. Of great interest, a newly recognized MHC "HLA-G associated haplotype" has been suggested to be independently protective for MS.

MS is not a simple hereditary disease, but it is more common in families of MS patients. Genome-wide screening in increasingly larger populations of patients continues to more clearly identify candidate genes for MS. Continued research into different forms of MS (clinical phenotypes) may identify genes (genotypes) that correlate with the disease if study populations are "homogeneous" enough and sufficiently large. Examination of specific gene functions will be the key to understanding their functional role.

Karen's comment:

My two sisters and I are often mistaken for triplets. We have statistically the least likely genetic composition that could result from our parents. Our tall, dark brown-eyed, brunette mother often called the three of us short, blue-eyed, blond daughters her "recessives!" My youngest sister has two daughters who also resemble us. There is a lot of immune-based illness in our family, including diabetes and allergy. When one sister had a ringing in her ear and migraines and a niece had unexplained falls, we held our collective breath until MS was ruled out for each of them. So far, I am the only one in my family who has been diagnosed with MS; however, I qualify this with "so far," as it is a concern that we cannot ignore.

50. Will my children get MS?

Children of parents with MS have an increased risk of developing MS. This chance is relatively small, however. Many years ago, studies in Minnesota established that the risk for children born to a mother with MS is

20 to 40 times higher than for the general population, and that female children have twice the risk as male children. However, these children will be under greater surveillance than members of the general population, and a diagnosis of MS is less likely to be missed. In other words, parents and other family members are not likely to ignore symptoms of milder illness. The risk in the general population is quite small, and even when an elevated risk is present, it corresponds to small percentages of affected persons. At present, one of 260 women in Minnesota who reach the age of 40 will be diagnosed with MS. This rate is similar to the risk for white women in Key West, Florida, the southernmost city in the continental United States.

Studies in Canada suggested that parents with the DR-2 gene (DR1 1501b) have an even higher risk of transmitting the probability of MS to their children than had been thought previously. It is clear from these studies that mothers have the greatest risk of passing on an increased risk of MS to their children, with girls possessing the DR-2 gene having the greatest risk. Care must be taken before extrapolating these observations to other populations, however. For example, the DR-2 gene is rare in Cuban Americans, yet MS is relatively common in this population. The population of patients with MS in Sardinia, Italy, has been studied intensively, and they too, appear to have different genes that correlate with their risk of MS. Siblings are reportedly 10 times more likely to develop MS than the general population. It is probably more correct to say that their risk of being diagnosed is 10 to 20 times greater.

Genes are the smallest bits of DNA that can pass on a hereditary characteristic to a child.

51. What are genes? Which genes cause MS?

Genes are the smallest bits of DNA that can pass on a hereditary characteristic to a child. They are located almost exclusively in chromosomes that are contained in the nucleus in the center of every cell in the body. Genes related to energy production are present in the **mitochondria**. Mutations are changes in the structure of the DNA that often alter the normal function of that gene. For those readers interested in the details of genes and their function, reviews of the subject can be found in the *Scientific American* journal and in encyclopedias.

Although there are probably no "MS genes" as such, MS patients have certain genes more commonly than other people do. The best known of these genes that occur more often in MS are members of the major histocompatibility complex (MHC) loci located on chromosome 6 at a point on the short arm of the chromosome at location number 21 (**Figure 7**). You may have heard of these

Mitochondria

The cells' power sources. These structures usually are rod-shaped but can be round. They have an outer membrane that limits the organelle and an inner membrane thrown into folds from projecting inward (i.e., "cristae mitochondriales").

Causes of Multiple Sclerosis

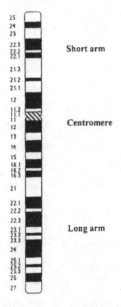

Figure 7   Drawing of chromosome 6 from the Human Genome Project. This drawing represents one of the pair of chromosomes. A chromosome has two arms or telomeres, a short arm and a long arm. There is a numbering system which starts at the centromere, the place where the telomeres join. Note the short arm (above) and also note position 21. This region (21) contains the "major histocompatibility (MHC)" genes: HLA-A, HLA-B, and DR. Many genes concerned with immune function are present in this region of chromosome 6. Collectively, genes of this part of the human genome have the highest rate of genetic mutation compared with any other part.

genes in relationship to organ transplantation; however, the majority of genes that play a role in immune function and autoimmunity are also found in this location. Four gene loci (locations) are especially important in relation to MS: A, B, C, and D. The "A" locus is a gene that codes for the MHC "class I protein"; it is the actual immune response gene for antibody production. The "DR" gene (at the D locus) is an immune response gene that codes for the MHC "class II protein," which plays a central role in cell-mediated immunity. These reactions principally involve monocytes and CD4 lymphocytes. Although the B locus is near the D locus, its role is not well understood. Many additional genes in this region of chromosome 6 are involved in immune reactions.

Mutations tend to occur at a higher rate in the MHC region than in the rest of the human genome. Several mutations or alterations in this region that are more common in MS have been identified. Minimal changes in gene structure, or even location, are sometimes referred to as **polymorphisms**. As you have undoubtedly heard, the Human Genome Project has recently deciphered the human genetic code, although many details regarding genes remain to be discovered. The Human Genome Project is presently looking for a pattern of single-nucleotide polymorphisms (SNPs)—that is, a "signature group of gene alterations." Once an individual SNP is identified, a search for the identity and function of the actual gene follows. A large number of SNPs are now known to be associated with a predisposition to MS, and others have been established as playing a role in Crohn's disease, another autoimmune illness. Separately, in a recent Swedish study funded by the Montel Williams Foundation, the MHC2TA gene (a "transactivator" gene at the MHC region) was shown to be associated with increased susceptibility to MS and

Polymorphisms

Referring to genetic polymorphisms, meaning many forms or shapes indicating the presence of mutations, chromosomal breaks, and transpositions.

rheumatoid arthritis. It is hoped that the identification of specific genes predisposing individuals to MS will eventually lead to preventive strategies.

A new field of epigenetic research has also emerged that has implications for MS. Approximately 700 small bits of genetic material called microRNAs have been identified through such study. They can modify the translation of the genetic of certain genes. The relationship of these molecules to MS is being investigated at present.

52. Is there a genetic reason why some people have severe disease?

In all probability, genetic factors explain why a very small percentage of patients develop very severe disease. Thirty-five years ago, a Danish group in Copenhagen found that when they tested MS patients who had suffered this rapidly progressive malignant disease, the majority of them had both the B-7 and DR-2 (DR1 1501b) genes, as discussed in Question 49. It is now known that the gene for **tumor necrosis factor**, which is a principal factor in damaging myelin, is contained within this region and that there are more active mutations of these genes in some MS patients than in normal individuals. The extension of the Human Genome Project, it is hoped, will extend these findings and shed further light on these genetic associations with severe disease. New specific therapeutic interventions may then follow.

Tumor necrosis factor

A principal factor made by macrophages that damage myelin.

OTHER FACTORS

53. I read that toxins can cause MS. Is this true? Can I be detoxified?

When people thought about toxins in the past, they usually referred to mercury, lead, arsenic, antimony, and other metals. Nowadays, insecticides are more often considered as potentially injurious. Hydrocarbons, poly-chlor-vinyls (PCVs) used in the manufacture of certain plastics, and other organic compounds are also topics of conversation and speculation regarding their impact on myelin and nervous system disease in general.

In fact, many potential toxins exist in our environment, although federal agencies and groups within our society are making progress in reducing our exposure to these agents. Problems caused by lead, mercury, and arsenic are real but do not appear to be issues that are especially relevant to MS patients. Few facts are available as to how much these toxins affect normal persons in the concentrations encountered in the environment, let alone how they may impact patients with MS. Indeed, there are more myths than facts regarding the role of toxins in health and disease.

Dental amalgam

The material dentists used for dental repairs (dental fillings).

One continuing concern is whether mercury in **dental amalgam**—the material used in dental fillings—is a health issue for MS. Although industrial mercury pollution was a major health problem in Japan and elsewhere, mercury in dental amalgam is a very different issue. There are inconsequential differences in serum and tissue levels of mercury in MS patients as compared with persons without this disease. No differences have been found in urinary excretion of mercury in MS patients. Moreover, in studies of edentulous (lacking teeth) MS patients who had never had any dental repairs, these individuals had higher levels of mercury simply because they consumed more fish. Thus there is no medical justification for removal of amalgam dental fillings from MS patients.

Likewise, the concept of "detoxification" has no place in the management of MS. Increased excretion of metals after "chelation" with drugs does not mean toxic levels were present in the person prior to chelation. Put simply, many of the measurements reported by laboratories are unreliable. Hair analysis is preferred to calculate levels of toxins present in the human body, but hair from the head is not suitable. Slow-growing hair such as pubic hair is the only appropriate specimen. Most patients, and some physicians, are unaware that chelating agents are themselves quite toxic and should be avoided, especially in treating MS patients! The bottom line is that there is no role for chelation therapy in MS.

54. Why do veterans have more MS?

The epidemiologic analysis of veterans' records for MS was not based on any evidence that veterans had an increased risk of MS, nor has any evidence been accumulated showing that military service increases the risk of MS. Certainly, there are abundant data showing that stress affects health in a variety of ways. Thus stress may be a factor in precipitating MS in the same ways in military life as in civilian life. However, the subject of military service, exposure to toxins peculiar to military life, and an increased risk of MS has not been the specific target of any prospective studies.

55. Can stress cause MS?

Stress has been shown to be an aggravating factor in MS but not a causal factor. More than 30 years ago, in conjunction with McGill University's Department of Psychiatry in Montreal, the author's research group found that major life stress (such as death or serious illness in a child or other family member, marital discord, and loss of employment) was three to four times more common in MS patients than in medical patients who had been referred to psychiatrists for psychiatric

Stress has been shown to be an aggravating factor in MS but not a causal factor.

consultation and care. Moreover, this stress was temporarily associated with relapses. Major life stress was also two to three times more common in the medical patients requiring psychiatric care than those not in need of psychiatric help.

Our finding that there is an association between stressful life events and attacks of MS has since been confirmed and extended in a number of studies in the United States and Canada. The most impressive was a San Francisco study showing that MS patients have new brain lesions detected in MRI brain scans more frequently when confronted with acute stress. A surprising finding was that "hassles"—those more minor irritations that just will not go away—were also associated with an increased risk of new brain lesions.

Certainly, there is a need for further scientific study of the biological consequences of stress and autoimmune disease. Such studies could lead to useful therapeutic interventions.

56. Can accidents bring on attacks of MS?

There is relevant history behind the issue of trauma and the risk of attacks, or the onset, of MS. The great Dr. Douglas McAlpine achieved international recognition for his specialization in MS at the Middlesex Hospital in London. Among his many original observations, he was the first to recognize that physical trauma increased the risk of MS exacerbations.

After moving to Montreal from Boston in 1971, I had the good fortune to work with my esteemed colleague, J. Bertrand R. (Bert) Cosgrove, at the Montreal Neurological Institute (MNI) at McGill University. He had been trained in neurology at the National

Hospital at Queen Square in London and with Dr. McAlpine. At that time, I was introduced to the reality of the clinical problem of MS.

We saw large numbers of MS patients, and Dr. Cosgrove introduced me to a myriad of less commonly recognized issues that patients with this disease confront. Dr. Cosgrove was especially interested in—and introduced me to—the issue of factors that increase the risk of exacerbations of MS. He pointed out that these factors included pregnancy, infection, burns, electric shock, stress, and surgical or accidental trauma.

Dr. Cosgrove emphasized that trauma, whatever the cause, was inevitably associated with emotional stress. With Dr. Lucien Gratton, a French psychopharmacologist and psychiatrist, we prospectively studied stress and found a strong association between stress and new attacks of MS. Dr. Cosgrove attributed the first recognition of these aggravating factors to Dr. McAlpine.

Despite the observations of McAlpine and Cosgrove, the relationship between trauma and onset or worsening of MS is considered to be unproven by some. Physicians of limited experience particularly echo this view. The critics are correct when they point out that this issue has not been studied scientifically. In the original observations, McAlpine did review his detailed clinical records retrospectively and did report a doubling of the risk of an attack of MS in association with surgery or other trauma. He pointed out that this relationship appeared to hold true even for dental extraction. In fairness, McAlpine's records were recorded and collected prospectively; in a more modern sense, they represented a database recorded on paper.

In contrast, Cosgrove observed that certain traumas were associated with greater risk than others. Importantly, accidents and surgical trauma similarly are associated with psychological stress. It is difficult, in most situations, to separate the physical from the psychological component in accidents and to elucidate their individual contributions in this regard. If this is true, how can the relationship be explained? Tissue trauma necessarily activates the immune system, which might reasonably lead to an increased risk of an attack of autoimmune disease in genetically predisposed individuals. It is likely that this reaction might serve to make a minor attack more clinically apparent.

PART FIVE

Living with Multiple Sclerosis

Now that I have been diagnosed with MS, how do
I learn to cope with this disease?

How does MS affect sexual function and fertility?

I'm having trouble coping with this diagnosis.
Should I seek professional counseling?

More . . .

Cerebrospinal fluid (CSF)

Fluid produced by the choroid plexus within the brain. It is located in the ventricles and surrounds the brain and spinal cord.

Syphilis

An infection caused by *Treponema pallidum*. Syphilitic infections are similar in type to infections caused by tuberculosis, but are potentially more serious. One type (meningosyphilis, meaning "vascular syphilis") can cause small strokes and its manifestations may resemble MS.

Systemic lupus erythematosus (SLE)

A chronic inflammatory autoimmune disorder that may affect many organ systems, including the skin, joints, and internal organs. The disease may be mild or severe and life-threatening.

Hypothyroidism

A disease of the thyroid associated with decreased secretion of thyroid hormone.

57. Now that I have been diagnosed with MS, how do I learn to cope with this disease?

Over the last four decades, as I have dealt with persons diagnosed with MS in my own practice, I have learned that each person reacts somewhat differently to a new diagnosis of MS. In many patients, the diagnosis is welcomed as an explanation for an event or events affecting their health that had previously remained unexplained. Others anticipated the diagnosis on the basis of life experience (the experience of a friend, relative, or celebrity dealing with MS). In some cases, surfing the Web or reading provided some insight into the illness. However, many come to MS centers for a "second opinion" because of an uncertain prior diagnosis.

The first step in dealing with MS is acceptance of the diagnosis (i.e., what does the diagnosis mean?). A diagnosis may be easy for the neurologist to make, but the affected person may not react positively or may even be suspicious about the seeming ease of establishing the diagnosis. Obviously, the confidence in the physician is a prerequisite in accepting the diagnosis. Although physicians other than neurologists may suspect the diagnosis, *the diagnosis of MS must be made by a neurologist.* It is also assumed that appropriate clinical neurologic examinations and tests such as MRIs of the brain and the spinal cord, **cerebrospinal fluid (CSF)** examination, and certain blood work will be performed and the results reviewed. These tests are usually needed to eliminate other diseases from consideration. Illnesses that can sometimes mimic MS, such as **syphilis, systemic lupus erythematosus (SLE),** and vitamin B_{12} deficiency, must be ruled out. Occasionally, patients will have MS as well as another disorder. One of the most common additional conditions found in MS is **hypothyroidism**. The presence of hypothyroidism does not rule out MS.

In actuality, the presence of this second autoimmune disease is supportive of the MS diagnosis.

An important practical point is that until the patient readily accepts the diagnosis, any decision regarding therapy has to be considered a tentative or temporary decision. The evidence is clear that *early treatment in MS is more effective,* and that withdrawal of treatment seems to precipitate additional (rebound) attacks in some people. Despite the importance of initiating treatment, some patients cannot readily accept the diagnosis and need assistance in dealing with the realities of their disease. The classic book *Denial of Illness* was based on the author's (Dr. Weinstein) experience with MS patients in a New York City MS clinic. It was the difficulty of MS patients in accepting the diagnosis and the implications of such a diagnosis that led to his classic publication. Denial of illness is not uncommon in young adults, but it seems to occur disproportionately more often in persons with MS.

A patient may accept the authority of the diagnosing neurologist without question, but in these times, this kind of "blind faith" is somewhat unusual. It is important that patients who are faced with the pronouncement of a diagnosis of MS are able to discuss the basis of the diagnosis and communicate with their neurologist. Most patients ask the questions posed in Part One of this book, such as "What is MS?" Although we know a great deal about the disease process in MS, we do not know the cause of MS (any more than we know the cause of cancer). Even so, in today's world, every new treatment is based on theories of how drugs interact with one or more steps in the disease process in MS. The results of these trials, regardless of a positive or negative outcome, provide new and better understanding

The evidence is clear that early treatment in MS is more effective, and that withdrawal of treatment seems to precipitate additional (rebound) attacks in some people.

Living with Multiple Sclerosis

of MS. With the great progress that has been made in the last 20 years, clarification of each step of the pathogenesis of the disease process will likely be accomplished and accepted in the near future.

Karen's comment:

The coping takes time. Sometimes it's just "fears and tears." The process is not a straight-line forward trajectory, and it requires more of me than I knew I had or sometimes have. My friends and family can be helpful but they have their own coping to do and sometimes are catching up with my changes as well as what is going on in their own lives. There are many frameworks to help people cope with a situation like MS. For myself, there have been three distinct phases of coping that I label "AAA": Accepting, Asking, and Advancing.

Accepting. I have MS. Almost as an echo to what Dr. Sheremata describes in his response to this question, when I first went to him and he confirmed I had MS, I realized that I had been secretly hoping he would not. When he was steadfast in the diagnosis of MS, I began to try to adjust. My second visit to Dr. Sheremata was equally jarring. Confident that I had accepted my new reality and adjusted my professional life accordingly, I explained to him I realized MS would prevent me from continuing my work as a law professor, so I was now volunteering to work as a support for lawyers and others trying to help overturn death penalty cases and had started slowly with a case for a young woman unjustly incarcerated with a double life sentence. I recall Dr. Sheremata gently noting that I was not really reducing my workload, stress, or expectations. That was when it hit me—this was not a brief time out or time off slight tweaking adjustment: MS was my new full-time job.

Acceptance also means acknowledging loss—of the me I knew and expected, friends, spontaneity, and being able to plan. Or as my friend Mary Ann put it, all the pictures in my future photo albums now looked different. It means giving up on some dreams and letting go of tangible and intangible remnants of the old me. It took me 5 years to finally throw away my law school course lecture notes and 8 years to give away law books that were already 3 years out of date. In the sixth year after I was diagnosed with MS, I gave my high heels to the woman who we were able to help release from prison. She had my size feet and when I sent them to her, I wrote her that I had saved them for when I walked "normally" or she walked freely.

Asking. *This phase involves learning to, whom to, what to, and when to ask for help. I used to think, with the grace of God, I could do it all. I never could before, and now I really can't. I am a very private (at least before contributing to this book) and independent person. However, as I balance and choose between help and independence, need and want, staying in the world and isolation, and safety and danger, I have to ask for help.*

Most people want to help. Some people we pay to care for me and our home. Others are volunteers. In both groups, I find an abundance of giving. Not everyone can or should help with everything. What seems to work best is to encourage people to say "no" when they mean it and "yes" when they mean it. Those who are helpful don't realize how their seem-ingly small action is such a gift. For instance, the UPS deliv-ery person brings packages inside when I can't move easily; the talented handyman brings me coffee; the cleaning lady folds clothes so even my husband's favorite "ratty red" T-shirt looks like designer clothing; and friends provide meals, untangle knitting messes I get into, learn to give me shots, and keep me company even when I simply lie on the floor.

Some people intuitively know or figure out what to do to help. One friend who did not at the time know much about MS or my tastes came for an afternoon to keep me company.

She brought six kinds of ice cream to allow for all possibilities: sugar-free; fat-free; dye-free; caffeine-free; dairy-free; and, what we ate the most of, the not-free-of-anything kind. But I can't expect anyone to read my mind. I relate to a character in a book by Elizabeth Berg who is in an iron lung; she explains to her teenage daughter that the hardest part of her life is, in essence, always having a glass of water at the temperature someone else decides to bring it. I have learned that it helps to be as specific as possible as to exactly what I need and what I want—but it is hard to not feel demanding or ungrateful for asking for the "water" at the desired temperature My father is my primary "caregiver" when my husband is away. So we have communication issues that are not just MS grounded but also normal parent–child and male–female focused. For example, when he grocery shops for me, he tries to tell me that cream of tartar is the same thing as tartar sauce. It also applies to emotions: When I cry or am sad, my father asks me, What is it again that he is supposed to do? My response is the thing that is the best help in most of my day is to just be with me.

Usually when I need or want help, it is not an emergency or dire situation, but rather involves the mundane activities that are part of daily life. I prefer to do many of them alone but can no longer do so safely. So I have choices: forgo the activity, modify it, or have a "spotter" at the ready. For example, it is not safe for me to shower alone; however, it is an activity that I need to do, and my husband often travels. So when I shower, I have a friend come over, I call someone when I get in and when I get out, or I have someone on the speakerphone. My sister works nearby as a CPA. I know if I want to shower during tax season, she can be found at her desk at all hours, and is happy to have me on the speakerphone in the background while she works and I shower. One time, upon stepping out of the shower, I jubilantly announced, "I am out. I am clean. I am wet, and I am naked." After a pause, I heard discreet coughing in the background, and my sister said, "And you are also on the speakerphone in our conference room." I have not visited her at work since.

Advancing. *Recently my husband and I moved to Princeton, New Jersey. This is our third time to live there. It is where we grew up, lived during the years just prior to and just after my diagnosis, and now live again after a 6-year absence. This literal return is helpful for perspective. Independent of my MS, friends and places have grown, grown up, and grown apart. Friends from "before MS" have had to learn what our new MS life is like. We need to help them help us by explaining what MS is (the first edition of this book was a good educator) and giving out my emergency contact information.*

During each of our adult chapters, we spent time looking for housing. This time, our criteria were so very different from before. Because I no longer drive, I wanted to be able to walk to places and/or be accessible so that others could visit me easily. The significant costs associated with my care and my not earning an income changed our budget. Because some days I can't climb stairs and some days I am alone part or all of the day, we needed one-story living or a place with an elevator or elevator-able. These criteria eliminated almost every one of the 400-plus housing options we saw. Sometimes we would see our "dream home" and be tempted to think backward and not with present and future realities. When we began to think that our only option was to pitch a tent in our friends' yard, my husband put a note in the mailboxes of four places we knew could work but were not on the market. We received a response from an owner of a newly built duplex with an elevator, located one block from the town square. We looked at the property for 15 minutes and 3 weeks later we moved in. I have looked more carefully at a pair of shoes than this home before owning it! But God's providence, coupled with a very helpful mortgage officer, a seller who is a medical person and a person of faith, friends, a cabinet maker whose wife has MS, and many others, all helped us make this move forward.

58. What do I need to know now that I have been diagnosed with MS?

You do not need to know how to make a watch to read time. In other words, it is not so important to understand every aspect of the MS disease process as it is to know that the vast majority of patients with MS will have the disease throughout their lifetime. It has been accepted that patients with MS will almost certainly have new symptoms along with relapses of old symptoms, with attacks tending to decrease in frequency and severity over the years. The interval between these attacks cannot be predicted with any accuracy, but most MS patients have an attack frequency ranging from one attack in 4 years to two or more each year.

Notably, in recent studies conducted at the University of California at San Francisco, half of the patients placed on one form or another of interferon-beta became relapse-free. This outcome is remarkable given the limited period of the study. Obviously, longer-term studies are needed to confirm this observation. Of great potential importance is that the finding that the relapse-free state appeared to have been predicted by the finding of specific genetic responses turned on by injection of interferon-beta. Clearly, the field of pharmacogenetics (genetic study of drug responses in humans and other animals) appears to hold great promise for selecting drugs for MS patients in the future. These types of studies are currently under way for low-dose interferon-beta-1a (Avonex) and Copaxone (in an NIH-sponsored study) as well as for many other agents not yet on the market.

For some patients, there is a tendency over a period of time to develop some disability. This is more serious when disability progresses between attacks and is the basis for making a diagnosis of secondary progressive disease (discussed in Part Three of this book). A recently published study of the natural course of MS in patients at the Mayo Clinic found that, on average, no statistically significant progression of disability occurred over a period of 10 years. However, 30% of these untreated patients did experience progression of disability. This kind of information is important to consider in making therapeutic decisions. Importantly, a variety of treatments for MS have been shown to affect virtually every type of disease that we recognize as MS (as discussed in Part Six of this book).

59. So many people want to be helpful, but I'm feeling overwhelmed and am not sure whether the information I am getting is correct. Where should I go for help?

The understanding, experienced physician is sufficient to meet the needs of most patients with MS. Often, the most important step is a matter of sweeping away unfounded fears and false conclusions about the disease and the effects of the disease on function. Friends and families are important to patients and often provide wonderful support, but the information that they have is not always correct or reasonably up-to-date.

Physicians knowledgeable about MS are the best sources for help. National Multiple Sclerosis Society support groups—if directed by professionals—can be of great help. The MS Society Web page (www.nmss.org) has current and up-to-date information as well as links to other sources of information. Even so, the personal

Physicians knowledgeable about MS are the best sources for help.

physician or neurologist is still the best conduit for information relevant to the patient. Physicians often encounter patients (and sometimes their immediate family members) who, when coached to ask appropriate questions, spill out baseless perceptions that severe disability such as paralysis and sexual dysfunction occurs often and early in this illness. Each of us has our own particular set of fears when it comes to how an illness will impact us. Doctors and nurses affected by illness are no exceptions.

Karen's comment:

To paraphrase Montel Williams, "They don't know what causes it; they don't know how to cure it; so it is up to you to decide how to treat your MS." I do decide how to treat my MS. However, after I use all my tools—research, prayer, list making, and more research—I still need advice from the medical professionals. I have an MS neurologist, a general practitioner, and various other specialists. They are all part of my MS decision-making process because MS is finely balanced by and disrupted by medications and changes in my environment and body. Things that seem straightforward or completely unrelated to MS may affect MS and require input from the neurologist.

As is evident from this book, my neurologist is Dr. Sheremata. Obviously, he is intelligent and cares about patient concerns. What may not be as apparent from the book and is important to me in choosing a physician are the "little things" that give me confidence in his advice and help. For example, Dr. Sheremata acknowledges it when he does not know the answer to one of my many questions and then tries to find answers; he listens to me and communicates with us via phone or email when we cannot be present geographically; he allows for positive outcomes even if they are unlikely; and he gives patients the ultimate choice unless he disagrees strongly with their decisions. In subtle ways, he also tends to my family and friends who are affected by my MS. I cannot imagine that I could get better care or caring from anyone else for my MS.

The non-MS doctors I go to are also good resources for help and advice related to my MS. Sensitivity to understanding that their specialty area of practice affects my MS demonstrates reliability for questions I have about MS. Further, it is a help when physicians creatively apply their specialty to MS-related problems. For example, I have gone to Dr. Selesnick (who is also the team doctor for the Miami Heat basketball team) for muscle and orthopedic issues. He performed a procedure on my shoulder that required 15 minutes of general anesthesia. Dr. Selesnick researched the issues involved with MS and anesthesia, and confirmed that the anesthesiologist had also done so. When he sent me for physical therapy for "foot drop," he did not prescribe a foot brace; instead, the aim was for me to be able to stand on one foot on a trampoline and catch a ball. I can't do that on all days, but it gave me a perspective to apply to other areas of my illness—to set a goal of living and not just bare existing or mere functioning. Of course, there are realities and limits; I don't think either of us expects that the Heat will be recruiting me anytime soon.

*With all physicians we ask for help, honesty is critical. The doctor I go to the most frequently is my general practitioner/endocrinologist/gynecologist doctor. His name is self-descriptive—Dr. Goodman. He is a good man. In the 20 years I have been a patient, he has managed my myriad of issues including hormones, cancer, and now MS. During my first appointment with him, he told me I would never have children and it was likely that I had **osteoporosis**. I had been to several doctors and none had told us this. He was the doctor who noticed I did not have an inner ear virus and sent me to a neurologist immediately, which led*

Osteoporosis

Porous bone; a disease characterized by low bone mass and structural deterioration of bone tissue, leading to bone fragility and an increased risk of fractures of the hip, spine, and wrist. Men as well as women are affected by osteoporosis, a disease that can be prevented and treated.

to my MS diagnosis. During those two particular visits, my life was altered in an instant in ways I hated. But amidst the pain and confusion, I am grateful that my doctor was clear, direct, and honest—and had a box of tissues on his desk.

60. I'm having trouble coping with this diagnosis. Should I seek professional counseling?

When faced with stress, it is difficult for us to understand and accept difficult issues such as a new diagnosis. Psychological counseling may help some patients with anxiety resulting from the stress related to their diagnosis. The inability to predict the course of MS, apart from a few generalities regarding the illness, sometimes detracts from any confidence patients might have in the treating neurologist. No neurologist can foretell the course for an individual patient, but MS takes on certain predictabilities in relationship to the course of illness. The reality of predictably effective, safe, and convenient therapy promises to take out much of the sting associated with accepting the diagnosis of MS. However, some patients will require the help of social workers, psychologists, or even psychiatrists to help them cope with anxiety precipitated by the new diagnosis.

Psychological counseling may help some patients with anxiety resulting from the stress related to their diagnosis.

61. Are there any MS "groups" that I can look into for additional help?

The National Multiple Sclerosis Society (NMSS) chapters and other groups have played an important part in education of patients and their families about MS. The NMSS chapters have regularly supported educational lectures for MS patients and their families. These sessions sometimes double as group therapy. When supervised by a professional, they are of real value to participants. Certainly, meeting other patients and exchanging experiences can help put the disease in perspective. It is important to recognize that the clinical course of illness varies greatly from one person to another. Young people may be intimidated when they meet severely affected individuals, regardless of their age or the duration of their illness. Therefore, potential participants in these sessions may wish to get more information about who will be present at a particular group session they are considering attending and whether it will be led by a knowledgeable professional.

The NMSS prints many helpful brochures, but the practice of mailing out dozens of brochures to unsuspecting newly diagnosed patients can be intimidating and, of course, wasteful.

Karen's comment:

I am not drawn to groups; usually I prefer a talk with God, a close friend, or a family member as a source of support. Nevertheless, I participate in MS support groups. I find them to be helpful as sources of information, and I hope I have been a source of support for other people. As with any group, there are dynamics and politics.

MS as a common bond makes it no more or less likely that I will necessarily like or want to spend time with a person. However, MS has created a connection with and introduced me to people whom I might never have known otherwise.

The people at the meetings, by and large, are there for positive reasons. They are generally well informed and well meaning. Additionally, there are the usual characters: the newly diagnosed person in denial who is sure it was a misdiagnosis and expects never to be at another meeting; the recently diagnosed person who expressed the same denial at a prior meeting; the person who is certain of and has all of the answers; the bee-sting aficionado; the lonely soul who has no other social contact; the nervous caregiver who eats cookies nonstop; and me. All of these people come together with stories that are unique, unnerving, empowering, irritating, enlightening, heartbreaking, tiring, and fascinating— MS in a nutshell.

MULTIPLE SCLEROSIS AND SEXUALITY

62. How does MS affect sexual function and fertility?

Patients and physicians in the past rarely discussed sexual function and performance despite its central role in life. This was especially true when illness other than heart disease was at issue. Sexual relationships are a major bond between married couples, and the new frankness about these issues particularly promises to benefit MS patients greatly. There are a number of pertinent issues in this regard, many of which are equally important to healthy persons.

Libido

Sexual interest or drive.

The most common sexual problem affecting both men and women in good health is a lack of **libido** (sexual interest or sexual drive). Psychological stress arising from interpersonal relationships and work is probably the most common single cause for this problem; it is obviously much more of an issue in young adults affected by a major health problem. The resultant uncertainties that naturally arise in these situations contribute to lack of libido greatly. The actual diagnosis of illness may induce acute stress, which can precipitate sexual difficulty or aggravate a preexisting sexual problem. In both men and women with MS, the loss of a feeling of well-being contributes to sexual dysfunction, whether accompanied by a depressed mood or not. Studies have shown that a caring, understanding relationship between the sexual partners is the single most important factor in maintaining good sexual health. It is important to be aware that the use of drugs for erectile dysfunction does not increase libido. Decision making in regard to changes of lifestyle and treatment for MS is an obviously important issue. Professional counseling is sometimes advisable.

Fatigue is a major symptom in MS and contributes to sexual dysfunction, just as it does in healthy men and women. Modification of lifestyle to conserve energy and the use of amantadine or other medications to increase energy are helpful. Amphetamine ("speed"), Ritalin, and cocaine are dangerous and should not be considered as options to eliminate fatigue. Patients should be cautious of the plethora of products flooding the health food market because some of these agents could actually contain harmful ingredients.

Karen's comment:

The topic of sex and MS has different components: how I feel about myself; how my husband feels about me; and how we feel together. These components naturally intertwine and interact. Before my diagnosis, I did not give my body much thought. I felt vibrant and was physically and sexually active, but my sense of myself was more cerebrally focused. I took my body, including sexuality, for granted, assuming that it would all just work without effort or intention. With my diagnosis and the effects of the steroids, I became almost fearful of my body—what was it going to do next? With time, fearless physical therapists, and the love of my husband, I have come to value and work hard on functioning physically. Furthermore, my view of myself sexually is independent of whether all of the parts of my body work on command and without pain. Rather, it depends on how I feel about myself, mind and body.

In the sixth grade, my husband wrote in my autograph book, "Have a great summer and please wear your sexy pink sweater often next year!" After 31 years of marriage, he still finds me sexually desirable; when I get out of the shower, he whistles. Nonetheless, MS has had an effect on how he relates to me sexually. Over the years, he has voiced concerns that he could hurt me, worries that I will get tired, and wonders whether I have physical sensations. Together, we manage MS and sex like other issues—with talking, laughing, and crying. My husband has many talents, but dancing and avoiding stepping on my feet is not one of them. I like to dance with him but between our respective challenges, it is not something we do often. When Tysabri came back to the market, I could not walk on my own, much less dance; however, my first infusion after the reintroduction of Tysabri seemed to me to be an event worth celebrating with a dance. My husband was reluctant to try this but I put on a favorite song, took off my clothes, and stood on my husband's feet. He was persuaded to dance.

Recently, I was on a panel focusing on issues of illness and caregivers. I relayed our feelings that we do not want my husband to be my full-time caregiver if we can find other good people to help me. Certainly, my husband does many caregiving tasks he had not done before my MS. Although he is trained to touch me to help with pain, stiffness, or spasms, we distinguish this "medicinal touch" from sexual touch. Both are done with love but have different mental and physical basis. Not only do we prefer for him not to do certain caregiving functions, by his own admission, he is much better at taking my clothes off than putting them on. He is totally inept at mascara, and pantyhose get him sidetracked! After I relayed this information to the audience, a petite grandmotherly woman raised her hand to speak: It was Dr. Ruth and she gave us her approval!

63. Do Viagra and other erectile dysfunction drugs help with impotence in MS?

The physical problem of erectile dysfunction is now openly discussed and is recognized commonly in otherwise healthy men. This change in the public attitude has helped men with MS accept this aspect of sexual function when it occurs and embrace the use of one of the approved drugs for erectile dysfunction. Viagra, Levitra, and Cialis appear to be at least as useful in men with MS as they are in otherwise normal men. Some studies have suggested that these drugs may also be helpful in women having difficulty achieving an **orgasm**. In any case, these medications should be used only under the supervision of a physician. Options to treat erectile dysfunction other than those just mentioned include drugs inserted into the **urethra** or injected directly into the penis, as well as implantable devices for males not responding to use of these medications. Such issues should be thoroughly discussed with physicians experienced with their use. However, surgery has special risks for men with MS.

Orgasm
Sexual climax.

Urethra
The anatomical tube connecting the bladder with the outside of the body. In the male, it extends to the opening in the penis.

Physical limitations affect men more than women in the sex act. The female partner can often compensate for movement difficulties if they limit sexual performance in her male partner. A willingness to experiment is healthy.

64. Are there treatments for loss of genital sensation?

A loss of sensation in the genital area can pose problems for both men and women with MS. Fortunately, such a loss of sensation in most patients is usually temporary. In men, the use of Viagra and similar drugs can, in part, overcome erectile dysfunction related to decreased sensation in some cases. Temporary or not, for many

Clitoral engorgement

Blood flow to the female sexual organ, the clitoris, that is associated with sexual excitement and results in clitoral enlargement (engorgement). It ultimately improves arousal and orgasm (sexual climax) in women.

Gynecologists

A physician who specializes in diseases that uniquely affect women.

Semen

The fluid portion of the ejaculate, consisting of secretions from the seminal vesicles, prostate gland, and several other glands in the male reproductive tract. Semen may also refer to the entire ejaculate, including the sperm.

Artificial insemination

Achieving pregnancy by artificial means. Most commonly, semen from a male donor is injected mechanically into the woman's vagina and/or uterus.

women, the use of vibrators can overcome the inability to achieve orgasm. Eros is a specially designed, commercially available device to enhance **clitoral engorgement** and provide stimulation for women who require it. It is important that women consult physicians who are knowledgeable in this area. Generally, **gynecologists** and sex therapists are better informed about these issues than most other types of physicians.

65. How can I get my wife pregnant if I am impotent?

Clinics dealing with spinal cord injuries, such as Veterans Affairs (VA) hospitals, are able to help with this problem. By using techniques that are similar to those employed in animal husbandry, **semen** can be harvested for successful use in **artificial insemination**. Personnel in spinal cord units at VA hospitals and universities should be contacted for help in this regard.

66. Can pregnancy bring on MS? What are the chances of an attack during pregnancy? Is it true that attacks are more severe after delivery?

Generally, women with MS feel better during pregnancy and have less likelihood of exacerbations of illness. During the first trimester of pregnancy the rate of attacks may be slightly increased, but during the second trimester there is a marked lowering of the risk of attack. By comparison, the third trimester is associated with a rising risk of exacerbation. In the 3 months after delivery, the risk of MS attacks is also high. A large French study showed that after delivery of the baby, the risk was increased by a factor of 3 for the first 3 months postpartum. Unexpectedly, the risk of exacerbations falls somewhat, to a twofold risk, for the next 33 months.

Earlier smaller studies in Minnesota had revealed an increased propensity to have exacerbations following pregnancy, whether or not the pregnancy went to term (lasted a full 9 months). In other words, termination of the pregnancy does not prevent the increased risk of exacerbation and worsened illness.

In summary, the chances of an MS attack during the first trimester of pregnancy are only slightly increased and fall substantially during the second trimester. However, there is an approximately 30% increased likelihood of an exacerbation in the third trimester of pregnancy and a marked increase in the 3 months after delivery. The numbers translate roughly into a 70% chance of exacerbation occurring in the 3-month post-delivery period.

Attacks postpartum tend to be more severe than average but, as at other times, the majority of MS attacks are not disabling. Treatment certainly can shorten these attacks. The advent of the new and more rapidly effective treatment, natalizumab (Tysabri, formerly referred to as Antegren), holds some promise for reducing this risk, but this drug has now been limited to patients who have failed standard treatment (interferon-beta or glatiramer [Copaxone]). The full effect of natalizumab in preventing attacks of MS is seen within 6 weeks after receiving the first dose. If indicated and used postpartum, this drug should not be given to the mother who is breastfeeding because of its potential presence in breast milk; its possible impact on the breastfeeding child has not been studied.

Karen's comment:

I have had many miscarriages and have no children. Before I was diagnosed with MS, I thought I felt good during

Living with Multiple Sclerosis

pregnancy because of emotions of joy and anticipation, and badly after a miscarriage, again because of emotions, albeit ones of grief and loss. Although emotions certainly played a part, I now understand that, as often is the case with MS, I had flare-ups after pregnancy.

•

Currently, I take hormone replacement therapy (HRT). I am fortunate to have an endocrinologist who is intelligent and who listens to patients. When I began HRT, he informed me about the many estrogens and progesterones. Finding a balance was a matter of trial and error—where error meant pimples and a desire to murder. The type and amount of each hormone affect my MS. I do better cognitively and physically when I take estrogen but not when I take progesterone. The particular "estrogen-only" pill I took was removed from the market for nonmedical reasons and to date there are no equivalents available. For several years my doctor creatively tried different compounds and delivery systems, each with varying success. Our most recent experiment is estrogen by injection; it is manufactured by the same international drug company that made the original estrogen pill I took before it was removed from the market. The vials of estrogen come via India; one order arrived wrapped in the Mumbai Sunday Times *and had a nonrequested Viagra pill included at no charge!*

67. Can pregnancy in a woman with MS harm the unborn child?

There is no evidence or expectation that MS directly affects the unborn child.

There is speculation that fertility is reduced in patients with MS and that the rate of spontaneous abortion is increased in the first trimester of pregnancy. There is no evidence or expectation that MS directly affects the unborn child. Based on the information collected in the North American Research Committee on Multiple Sclerosis (NARCOMS) database, the interferon-beta treatments for MS (Betaseron, Avonex, and Rebif) do appear to pose an increased risk of birth defects in the unborn child. Although the potential risk appears to be measurably lower for Copaxone, use of this drug during pregnancy cannot be recommended.

The increased risk of MS in the child is another issue that has already been discussed. This is a genetic issue and is unrelated to whether the mother was diagnosed prior to the pregnancy.

Living with Multiple Sclerosis

PART SIX

Treatment of Multiple Sclerosis

What are the treatments for MS?

Do "folk remedies," such as snake venom and bee venom treatments, work for MS?

How are MS attacks treated? Why are there different drugs to treat attacks of MS?

More . . .

68. What are the treatments for MS?

The last two decades have witnessed the approval of several drugs specifically for MS. Although used for exacerbations of MS for more than 20 years prior to Food and Drug Administration (FDA) approval and validation of its use in several studies (including a national trial reported in 1970), adrenocorticotrophic hormone (ACTH; Acthar Gel) was not approved by the FDA until 1978. It remains as the sole approved drug for treatment of MS exacerbations. In contrast, five injectable drugs have been approved to reduce the risk of exacerbations and disability within the last 17 years. Dalfampridine (4-amino-pyrine) has just been improved to "improve mobility." Finally, approval of two oral drugs that appear to be highly effective in reducing exacerbations and risk of disability is anticipated within the next year. We hope that additional oral agents will follow them to the market. Although these new oral agents are more effective than the interferon products, only fingolimod has been subjected to head-to-head comparisons with interferon-beta-1a. As always the risk–benefit balance must be weighed with these new agents. The more immunosuppressive the drug is, the greater the risk of infection and malignant complications is likely to be. Risk management (i.e., better follow-up safety monitoring) can be expected as a condition for approval of these drugs.

Symptomatic treatment does not alter the disease process but rather is aimed at relieving symptoms.

Treatments for MS may be classified into three categories: symptomatic treatment, acute relapse management, and treatment aimed at the reduction of the risk of relapses as well as disability.

Symptomatic treatment does not alter the disease process but rather is aimed at relieving symptoms. Treatment of relapses will usually reduce symptoms and the resultant disability associated with the relapse more quickly than would occur naturally, but it does not alter the disease process either. A reduction of relapses will, of course, reduce temporary disability associated with attacks but is most meaningful if it reduces the risk of disability.

Fatigue and urinary tract complaints are among the most common symptoms that MS patients experience that are amenable to treatment. Many disturbances of sensation are highly subjective symptoms. Not uncommonly, a feeling of numbness is present only when attention is focused on the particular complaint, and it does not interfere with daily activity. Painful sensations may be favorably affected by treatment. Generally, the more severe the pain, the more likely it will be alleviated by medication.

Narcotics are not indicated; indeed, they are contraindicated in MS. Marijuana and its purified psychoactive component, delta-9-THC, have failed to show objective benefit for pain and **spasticity** in studies; in our practice, we do not prescribe them for any MS patients. Drugs used in the management of **epilepsy** are the mainstay of pain management in MS, although other drugs may also be helpful in this regard. The manifestations of spasticity, such as stiffness and muscle spasms, can greatly benefit from treatment.

The approval of dalfampradine for MS to improve mobility was based on its documented ability to help patients walk short distances more quickly and, presumably, with less fatigue. This symptomatic treatment targets specific mechanisms that are impaired in MS.

Karen's comment:

The illegality, availability, and choice of treatments are very personal. When I was in college, I knew I wanted to

Narcotics

Drugs that produce morphine-like effects. This term is derived from the Greek word for "stupor," and originally referred to a variety of substances that dulled the senses and relieved pain.

Spasticity

Velocity-dependent increase in muscle tone.

Epilepsy

A brain disorder that occurs when the electrical signals in the brain are disrupted, leading to a seizure.

Treatment of Multiple Sclerosis

be a lawyer. At the time we had to sign something to be admitted to the bar that essentially asked you if you had taken any illegal drugs—so you could avoid taking the drugs or take the drugs and lie (compounding the error). My then-boyfriend (now my husband) can attest that in college, due to my desire to be a lawyer, I was vigilant about not taking drugs and even left parties when people were using drugs. I still am a lawyer. I still don't take illegal substances.

Despite my decision related to my own pain treatment, my horse is not as high as it may seem. I have gone to great lengths to secure legal medicines for myself and for others. For cognition, I have tried medicines on an "off-label" basis (i.e., use of an approved medicine for other than their intended indications). Further, I have tried medicine that was legally imported from other countries for my personal use—for example, when memantine was not yet available in the United States, the AIDS community dispensed it to people with a prescription from a New York City warehouse. As I describe later, I did take Tysabri after it was removed from the market until I ran out of it.

As for treatment that is not approved in the United States and is specifically prohibited, I understand that marijuana helps many people relieve pain they cannot get from other remedies. I also understand the desire to help loved ones who are in pain get relief by whatever means possible. I have a friend who is the wife of a rabbi and the daughter of a woman with MS who lives in the United Kingdom. A few years ago, her mother was coming to the United States for a visit and needed to have the pain reliever she is prescribed and takes in the United Kingdom: marinol (a pill form of cannabis). We convinced her that the sniffer dogs at the Miami airport were likely to identify her medicine as marijuana and illegal, and she should leave it behind. So we decided to get her some here. I began by calling a few people and put up with their mocking my claim that the marijuana was for a "friend's mother." We found out where we might obtain the drug/medicine after dark under a bridge in a particular part of town. Pleased at being able to help her mother, as we started off in her van. Fortunately, we stopped a moment and thought of the headlines: Rabbi's Wife, Mother of 7; Minister's Wife, Legal Ethics Professor: ARRESTED While Buying Drugs in Miami. So we abandoned our plan. Even more fortunately, we found an alternative—and legal—option for her mother.

69. Do "folk remedies," such as snake venom and bee venom treatments, work for MS?

Sir Augustus D'Este, a grandson of King George III of England, was the first person clearly known to have MS. The treatment he received, as revealed in his diary, was entirely symptomatic. We would not consider repeated **enemas** and bloodletting to be symptomatic treatment today. Unfortunately, many of the kinds of treatment that today's patients and their families embrace are just as rational as those that D'Este received.

MS treatment in the past was essentially symptomatic—that is, treatment aimed solely at alleviating specific symptoms or making patients feel better. Although that may sound good, it was not enough by itself. Treatments were not based on scientific study. Most were not effective, and some were harmful. Similarly, operators of health food stores today sell a large variety of unproven herbal remedies that they justify with unsubstantiated claims. By and large, the herbal preparations and most other preparations sold in such stores should be avoided.

Enemas

Liquids that are used to facilitate bowel evacuation; usually water- or oil-based materials. They are put into the rectum via an enema tube attached to a bag or other container.

Decades ago, as an intern, I was asked to deliver intravenous alcohol to a patient with MS. The prescribing neurosurgeon stated that he had just read a paper in a medical journal claiming a benefit from this form of treatment. Despite my reservations, I complied with the order. The patient became intoxicated but, nevertheless, felt that she had been helped. The neurosurgeon was embarrassed and abandoned this therapy. Later in my training, I was advised by Lord Brain, a famous British neurologist of the day, that "any drug that had been used for any therapeutic purpose had been tried on patients with MS." I have subsequently come to realize that he was not exaggerating. The major problem is not so much that these measures are unhelpful but rather that many of the treatments are potentially dangerous. Untested drugs, whether purified or in their crude state, should be viewed as potentially dangerous in their own right or by virtue of drug interactions.

Snake Venom

Several decades ago, a self-styled microbiologist in Florida presumed that if an animal (or human) recovered from a snake bite, that recovery occurred because of a biological reaction (perhaps an antibody) that eliminated the offending venom. He reasoned further that the response to snake venom (an antibody) could eliminate offending cross-reacting infectious agents such as poliovirus or toxins. He started giving injections of diluted venom to believers with a variety of illnesses, many of whom provided testimonials claiming improvement. When the serpentarium in South Miami that had provided the snake venom closed around 1980, the source of the venom disappeared, but the myth persisted. After examining many dozens of MS patients who had received venom over a period of years, I concluded that there was no evidence that they had

Untested drugs, whether purified or in their crude state, should be viewed as potentially dangerous in their own right or by virtue of drug interactions.

benefited from their experience, even though published research has revealed antiviral activity in the natural snake venom.

Bee Venom

Folk remedies are often applied with both great conviction and great ceremony. One such practice, which originated in the jungles of South America, involves applying bee stings for **arthritis**. Several years ago, a scientific study was carried out that initially seemed to confirm some benefit from this practice. Subsequently, purification of the venom was performed in an attempt to find a marketable product. This led to the finding of a single protein in the bee venom that was thought to be the active ingredient. Unfortunately, this purified protein failed to relieve arthritis, and scientific research was halted.

Claims that bee stings offer a therapeutic benefit for MS have no scientific basis, and no reputable pharmaceutical company is likely to pursue this issue. Moreover, this practice has a real potential to harm MS patients who are immunosuppressed from certain treatments such as steroids, azathioprine (Imuran), or methotrexate. There are tetanus spores in bee venom; in immunosuppressed patients, germination of these spores can lead to **tetanus**, which is potentially fatal. The only notable effects in MS patients that I have witnessed related to "bee sting therapy" have been allergic reactions complicated by serious deterioration, ending in death for a small number of MS patients. In my own practice, we have never used or recommended bee venom as a treatment for MS.

A word of warning: Any layperson can walk into a health food store and be met with multiple unfounded claims for products that can be obtained without a prescription. Buyer beware!

Arthritis
A term commonly used to describe joint disease causing pain. It should actually be reserved for inflammatory disease of joints, such as rheumatoid arthritis.

Tetanus
A potentially fatal illness produced by infection with the bacterium *Clostridium tetani,* most often complicating wound contamination. It is characterized by rapidly increasing stiffness and may lead to seizures and death.

70. Is there anything I can do about my overwhelming fatigue?

Effective treatments for fatigue are available. Amantadine is a drug that was approved more than 40 years ago to prevent and subsequently treat influenza; it has also been proven to be of benefit in reducing fatigue in MS. Drugs such as amphetamine and Ritalin have been used for this purpose as well, but none is as safe and as well tolerated as amantadine. Moreover, habituation to Ritalin and amphetamine occurs quickly. More recently, modafinil (Provigil), which was approved for management of narcolepsy, has been prescribed in MS and has shown limited effectiveness. Tolerance seems to develop quickly in some patients, and higher doses are often not well tolerated. Some patients do experience a sustained improvement. Importantly, this drug is relatively expensive.

The drug 4-amino-pyridine (dalfampradine) is a very old drug that has been compounded in pharmacies for many years. In frog spinal cord studies conducted many years ago, it was shown to have effects that should be helpful in MS. Preliminary studies by Dr. Floyd Davis, who did the frog studies in Chicago, then showed benefit in MS patients but 5% of patients had epileptic seizures shortly after starting the drug. An extended-release form of dalfampradine has been shown to be safe and effective in studies. It has just received FDA approval for use in MS based on trials that showed a reduction in the time required to walk a measured distance. This drug also seems to induce an improved sense of well-being and a reduction in fatigability. Users who might be tempted to buy dalfampradine from compounding pharmacies should be warned that the drug is very unstable and requires special formulation to prevent breakdown. The compounded formulations are "immediate-release" products and, if any biological activity is present, will carry the risk of inducing seizures.

Karen's comment:

My family and I refer to fatigue as "fat-goo" after a kind, but inexperienced nurse trainee who was unfamiliar with the word pronounced it the way it feels—like I'm trying to go through fat and goo to function. I am unable to will myself to do something that I feel I should otherwise be able to do. What I find most difficult about fatigue is managing it psychologically. I get tired of being tired. Sometimes I feel as if I should try harder to get "through the goo," but usually when I try this I end up falling, dropping something, and overloading cognitively. Then I have more to do when I am functioning again.

Fatigue is also hard on others psychologically. It is an invisible symptom—part of the "but you look so good" phenomenon. This is when well-meaning people will look at me and say to themselves or to me, "I would never know you had an illness; you look so good." While on one level it is flattering, mostly it is hard; they have no idea how hard it is to function and perform everyday tasks such as brushing my teeth, getting dressed, and sitting up in a chair—much less walking. I treat my fatigue with amantadine, caffeine (preferably Cuban colada), and sugar in a form that I can carry with me and take in small portions, such as M&Ms and jelly beans. Dr. Crayton has noted that caffeine has the benefits of being mostly affordable, has no insurance issues, and can be titrated .These "medicines" do not always get me through, but they help. The other remedy for fatigue is getting help—volunteer and paid.

During a long flare-up, we decided to hire an aide for 1 day a week. It was hard to take this step, but those around us expressed relief and voiced surprise that I had not done this earlier. I was blessed to find a nurse who is flexible and understands my situation. During bad days, she gets me up, does range-of-motion exercises, makes breakfast, and gets my medicine. On the good days, we have fresh-picked strawberries, deliver food to shut-ins, and run errands. When I told my family about hiring her, they were at first very defensive and felt that they should do these things with and for me. Now that time has passed, we all have experienced the benefit she gives us. I am more independent and physically safer. My family members have one day a week that they are not on-call and can relax knowing that I am with a great professional. It helps, and we are all less fatigued.

71. What can I do about getting rid of this stiffness in my legs? What is the best treatment for spasticity?

A feeling of stiffness often is symptomatic of spasticity, although it may occur for other reasons. If you have cramps in your calves, especially at night, the problem is probably spasticity, for which there are a number of different therapies. In contrast, if the feeling of stiffness is due to impaired sensation in the legs, these treatments will not help.

Runners and other athletes use stretching of muscles to relieve muscle cramps. Not surprisingly, the first proven approach to the treatment of spasticity consisted of stretching the affected muscles. In the last three decades, several drugs have been proven to be helpful, including Valium (diazepam, which was the first drug studied for this purpose), Lioresal (baclofen), and, most recently, Zanaflex (tizanidine). A single 5-mg dose of diazepam at night is often sufficient for milder forms of spasticity. It has the advantage of being very long acting. Thus, if the spasticity is not severe, a single dose at nighttime may be sufficient for the entire day.

Baclofen can be effective in cases of spasticity, but many patients do not get an effect that is proportional to the dose (that is, they have a poor dose-response). Actually, diazepam and baclofen have the same biochemical effect in the body that reduces spasticity. Usually there is no need to give additional daytime doses of diazepam. If 5- to 10-mg doses of diazepam cause excessive daytime sedation or if these doses are insufficient to control stiffness or muscle cramps, the use of baclofen or tizanidine may be necessary. Tizanidine is a newer drug that has the advantage of not trading spasticity for weakness. Unfortunately, it may produce drowsiness and intolerable dryness of the mouth. Baclofen and tizanidine can be used together for additional benefit. Tizanidine is not usually prescribed in combination with diazepam because of the probability of excessive sedation. Capsules of tizanidine are a newer timed-release form of this drug; they reduce the chances of sedation and, importantly, prolong its relatively shorter action. Another drug, dantrolene hydrochloride (Dantrium), is used infrequently for treatment of spasticity because of its potential liver toxicity.

Relief of spasticity can be a disadvantage to some patients if they use spasticity to help in standing and weight bearing. All of the drugs mentioned here as treatments for MS-related spasticity should be prescribed and monitored by a neurologist who can assess their effectiveness and modify doses or change the medication to the patient's advantage. Simply withdrawing an effective medication because of a side effect may not be a wise decision. Sedation can be a problem with all of the drugs

Treatment of Multiple Sclerosis

used, not just with diazepam. Continued use and slow rates of dosage increase can help avoid this issue.

Karen's comment:

Spasticity for me has ranged from slight stiffness to extreme stiffness that makes me look like a mechanical doll. In between the extremes is tightness. If I get into the wrong position, I require another person to "untangle me." The tightness can lead to rigidity, followed by an almost limpness as a result of exhaustion of the muscles involved. Sometimes there is a lot of pain; at other times it is painless.

There are many treatments for spasticity. Dr. Sheremata has remarked that only one mouse in the studies is as sensitive to these medications as I am. My first experience with baclofen left me so weak from one pill that I could barely sit up or function for 3 days; thus I have not retried it. When I took Tegretol, I threw up from each dose and felt very unlike myself—almost altered and distanced from my own being. So I have not retried it either. When I took Neurontin, I immediately threw up despite the minor dose.

During one severe episode of spasticity, we were reluctant to try medication. I spent 3 days stiff and in extreme pain. In desperation, my husband carried me into the swimming pool that we are fortunate enough to have in our backyard. My muscles relaxed, and I fell asleep in his arms. My husband is very intelligent; however, he had not thought through what to do in this circumstance: 2 A.M., holding a sleeping wife in a pool with no phone or book nearby. He lasted 3 hours and woke me with both of us resembling prunes! For the next few days, when I would start to stiffen up, I would get into the pool, and it would pass. After several nights of splashing, moans, and groans coming from our side of the fence, our neighbors finally got up the nerve to ask us what exactly we were doing in the middle of the night!

For more "normal" spasticity, I stretch at yoga class and ballet class. In addition, I have others stretch me: Professionals help two times a week, and my family is now trained at leaning, kneading, and pushing the various parts of me that need it. I am not always able to do the yoga or ballet, and sometimes, the most that I can manage is getting into a leotard (not an easy feat at my age in any event) and getting to class. Yet the training and muscle memory and the feeling of doing things for my body that are not strictly therapeutic or medicinal are very empowering. It stretches me to places I thought I would never go.

72. Is it true that baclofen can be injected? How does that work?

Baclofen can be injected to reduce spasticity, but it is only available for injection into the spinal fluid using an implantable pump. Direct injection into the spinal fluid is used only as a test to evaluate the patient's response before implanting the pump. This device allows the baclofen to be delivered into the spinal fluid continuously. This treatment, which is called **intrathecal** baclofen, is used only for patients with severe spasticity who cannot tolerate the side effects or do not benefit from oral baclofen. The injectable drug differs in its composition, making it more effective. Ordinarily, intrathecal baclofen is not considered in ambulatory patients. Pump implantation is best carried out in centers with experience in both placement of the pumps and management of MS patients.

Intrathecal
Inside the central nervous system.

73. Is it true that Botox injections can be used to treat spasticity?

Yes. Botox can be used to relieve spasticity. However, only neurologists or specialists in physical rehabilitation who are familiar with and experienced in both the use of this drug and the special problems that MS patients may encounter should use Botox. Generally, this drug is reserved for patients who have severe spasticity with early contractures in a single muscle group, such as the **gastrocnemius**, and who have failed management with stretching and the drugs previously discussed. Botox is not a panacea for the management of spasticity.

74. Why do some patients with MS become unable to urinate when they have to urinate all day and night?

Bladder function is complex. Emptying the bladder is the result of three parts of the bladder functioning in sequence. To empty urine from the bladder effectively, the bladder wall (the **detrusor muscle**) has to contract. When the pressure in the bladder has reached the right level, only then will the bladder neck relax normally and then the internal **sphincter** relax. If the external sphincter is relaxed, voiding will occur. Sometimes, early in the course of MS, the bladder may not contract normally, so that the sphincter does not relax, preventing the bladder from emptying. This is a so-called **hyporeflexic bladder**. Most bladders are actually hyperreflexic, and the patient feels the urge to urinate frequently, sometimes with a feeling of great urgency. At times, the bladder uncontrollably empties unexpectedly or prematurely, resulting in urinary **incontinence**.

Treatment of bladder dysfunction is usually directed at relieving symptoms and reducing the risk of infection. Ditropan (oxybutinin) and other similar **anticholinergic** drugs are the mainstay of the treatment of urinary frequency and urgency. Unfortunately, these drugs tend to produce dryness of the mouth. Often, patients prefer to use the drugs only at night to reduce wakening and risk

Gastrocnemius

The large calf muscle that pulls and keeps the foot down (plantar flexes the foot).

Detrusor muscle

The muscle of the urinary bladder that forms the actual storage organ and is the largest part of the bladder.

Sphincter

A circular muscle that constricts a passage, such as the urethra or the anus. When relaxed, a sphincter allows materials to pass through the opening; when contracted, it closes the opening.

Hyporeflexic bladder

Decreased bladder reactivity as defined by urodynamic testing in a laboratory.

Incontinence

Urinary incontinence; involuntary loss of bladder control.

of incontinence. These drugs can also be useful when patients with urinary frequency and urgency have to leave their homes. Urinary **catheterization** is sometimes necessary to achieve bladder emptying and can help prevent recurrent bladder infections and complicating kidney damage. If catheterization is recommended, it should be done regularly. All patients with such problems should be seen by an urologist who is familiar with these problems associated with MS.

TREATMENT OF MULTIPLE SCLEROSIS ATTACKS

75. How are MS attacks treated? Why are there different drugs to treat attacks of MS?

MS is characterized by unpredictable attacks of neurologic symptoms that vary greatly in type and severity. After being diagnosed, all patients are familiar with at least one symptom. They are concerned about recovering from the difficulty as soon as possible. Generally, recovery follows all attacks, whether treatment is given or not. The speed of recovery is the only predictable outcome that is affected by treatment.

If a patient cannot perform his or her responsibilities at home or at work, shortening these more severe attacks by using drugs would seem to be of paramount importance. At present, adrenocorticotrophic hormone (ACTH; Acthar Gel), also called corticotrophin, remains as the only FDA-approved treatment for attacks (relapses) of MS. Nevertheless, most neurologists prescribe either oral or high-dose intravenous steroids (methylprednisolone [Medrol®]) for exacerbations of MS. Some neurologists prescribe steroids as ongoing therapy for MS patients, even though there is no scientific basis for this practice. In addition, there are many potential side

Anticholinergic

A descriptor for drugs that block the effect of the hormone acetylcholine in the body. These drugs include atropine, scopolamine, and Ditropan. They slow the heart rate down, dry secretions, and reduce the contractions of the bowel and bladder. These drugs produce dryness of the mouth and constipation as common side effects.

Catheterization

Removal of urine from the bladder by means of a urinary catheter (tube).

MS is characterized by unpredictable attacks of neurologic symptoms that vary greatly in type and severity.

Treatment of Multiple Sclerosis

effects from chronic use of steroids. Steroids do reduce fatigue in MS patients and often induce a sense of well-being. Their many side effects, however, do not justify their use for those reasons.

One study did show accelerated recovery from attacks of optic neuritis after the use of high-dose intravenous (IV) methylprednisolone (Solumedrol). In contrast, oral steroids had no effect except to double the risk of relapse of optic neuritis as compared with IV Solumedrol. There often is a rapid response to either drug in patients with acute, severe relapses, but there are no good studies of IV Solumedrol versus ACTH or compared with higher doses of oral steroids in MS.

Progressive multifocal leukoencephalopathy (PML)

A serious infection of the brain that is caused by the JC papillomavirus.

Cataracts

Any opacification (loss of transparency) of the lens of the eye or its capsule. Cataracts are not considered significant if they do not interfere with vision.

Necrosis

Tissue death; a state of irreversible tissue damage.

The side effects of steroids include an increased risk of infection, including viral, bacterial, yeast, fungal, and parasitic infections. This risk also includes **progressive multifocal leukoencephalopathy (PML)**, which was reported to occur in two patients treated with Avonex and with Tysabri, and subsequently in 31 additional patients (out of more than 60,000 patients worldwide as of January 2010). Other complications of steroids include psychiatric problems, **cataracts**, osteoporosis, and ischemic **necrosis** of hips and other joints.

Steroids, including methylprednisolone, induce programmed cell death of cells in the body, not only in lymphocytes but also in neurons in the brain and the retina. Studies performed more than three decades ago have shown that corticotrophin has a powerful neuroprotective effect. This is yet another reason supporting the use of ACTH (corticotrophin) in MS. The search goes on for other neuroprotective agents that might have comparable or better effectiveness and fewer side effects.

Karen's comment:

To steroid or not to steroid? Dr. Sheremata is in the minority on this issue. However, I have followed his advice not to take the customary steroids and instead consider rest and ACTH. Despite the side effects of steroids that I experienced the only time I took them and the factual knowledge that we have about them, it has been hard not to take steroids when I have a flare-up.

When I have a flare-up, I will call or email Dr. Sheremata and ask him to remind us again about his view. The desire on my part and those around me is to do something to alleviate the flare-up. The fear, the lack of control, the symptoms themselves, and the uncertainty all make it difficult to take the rest approach and not to take the steroid approach. However, I have followed the rest regimen (as my family calls it "Dr. Sheremata medicine"), and I believe that I have recovered faster and stronger than if I had gone the steroid route. Furthermore, I do not have to recover from the steroids. Nonetheless, if and when I have my next flare-up, I imagine I will still re-ask the question. Perhaps this book should be titled 100 Times the Same Question About MS Is Asked!

76. What is ACTH?

Adrenocorticotrophic hormone (ACTH), also known as corticotrophin, is a hormone that is produced in the brain and is stored in the **pituitary gland**, which is situated at the base of the brain. This hormone is normally released in miniscule amounts during the early hours of the morning to stimulate the **adrenal glands'** production of steroid hormones. **Cortisol**, the active form of **cortisone**, is one product of ACTH stimulation. Dr. Leo Alexander began using ACTH as a treatment for MS more than a half-century ago at

Pituitary gland

An endocrine gland about the size of a pea that is located at the base of the brain. The pituitary gland secretes hormones regulating a wide variety of bodily activities, including trophic hormones that stimulate other endocrine glands.

Adrenal glands

Glands of internal secretion situated above the kidneys, and hence sometimes referred to as supra-renal glands. The cells of the cortex (on the outside of the gland) secrete cortisone and other steroid hormones that are important in the body's response to stress.

Cortisol

The primary steroid hormone (17-hydroxy-corticoid) produced by the adrenal gland. It is the biologically active soluble form of cortisone.

Cortisone

The stored form of cortisol produced by the adrenal cortex.

Harvard Medical School at the behest of Dr. George Thorn, who had studied adrenal function extensively. Dr. Alexander showed in a series of studies that it speeded recovery from MS attacks. After multiple studies in Europe showed benefit in shortening attacks of MS, a national double-blind, controlled study, published in 1970, proved that ACTH does, indeed, significantly speed the recovery for patients with acute exacerbations of MS.

Acthar Gel, the commercial product, was withdrawn from the market when Parke Davis stopped manufacturing many drugs a number of years ago. However, as a result of the efforts of the National Organization for Rare Diseases (NORD) and the National Multiple Sclerosis Society, as well as the recognition of the value of ACTH, Acthar Gel is again available. The intravenous form of Acthar is no longer available, and the synthetic form for intravenous use is in extremely short supply.

More than a quarter-century of research has shown that ACTH also has neuroprotective properties, although clinical neurologists are rarely aware of this fact. In recent scientific studies of experimental optic neuritis in rats, high-dose IV steroids were shown to actually induce the death of brain nerve cells. ACTH has the opposite effect: Its neuroprotective effect was established more than three decades ago.

77. Why aren't drugs used together to get a better effect?

ACTH and IV steroids are not ordinarily used together. However, high-dose IV steroids (in 1-g daily doses) theoretically could be used for a 3- to 5-day period in patients who have especially severe attacks to reduce swelling in the optic nerve or spinal cord, with ACTH added to maintain adrenal function (because steroids suppress the adrenal glands), thereby obtaining the benefit of the other actions of ACTH. This would also provide the neuroprotective effect of ACTH.

Although you may ask, "Why not continue the high-dose IV steroids?"—it is important to recognize that high-dose steroids damage myosin, which is the main protein in muscle that is responsible for muscle contraction. Prolonged use of IV steroids may result in serious muscle damage, sometimes referred to as "intensive care unit paralysis." This is yet another reason why it is unwise to continue high-dose steroids for longer periods.

Prolonged use of IV steroids may result in serious muscle damage, sometimes referred to as "intensive care unit paralysis."

78. How do ACTH and steroids compare as treatments for MS?

Very few studies have addressed this issue—that is, treatment comparisons—because of the absence of commercial interest in their outcomes. In fact, the NIH supported the national study of ACTH, the results of which were published in 1970. The more recent NIH-sponsored study of optic neuritis was the first attempt to compare oral versus IV steroids and placebo. This study failed to show any benefit from oral steroids; indeed, use of oral steroids increased relapses.

A small study in England revealed similar outcomes obtained with IV steroids and ACTH; however, the numbers of patients were very small, and the study consequently suffered from problems in statistical analysis of the results (a Type II error). Essentially, a Type II error occurs when a study compares two treatments but fails to enroll a sufficient number of patients to take each of the treatments. The benefits may seem not to differ, but the conclusion that benefits from the two drugs are the same is not valid.

A number of other small studies have been carried out, from which it is not possible to draw valid conclusions. Valid studies have to be large and, as a result, are very expensive to conduct.

79. Why should I take drugs that have side effects?

This is an excellent question. Although patients recover from attacks of MS with or without drug treatment, recovery is hastened with ACTH treatment.

In the 1970 ACTH national study, MS patients in relapse were all placed at rest hospitals. In this relatively small study, despite being hospitalized and benefiting from rest, actively treated patients receiving ACTH were significantly better after 1, 2, and 3 weeks of ACTH treatment compared with those receiving placebo injections. Although the patients had less disability at 4 weeks (2 weeks after termination of treatment) as compared with placebo recipients, the difference was not statistically significant. Other studies probably should have been done to answer questions about the effectiveness or particular doses of ACTH as well as questions related to dose forms (e.g., gel versus IV), but they were not. Despite their importance, it is unlikely that any such studies will be carried out on a significant scale anytime in the future.

It should be appreciated that physical rest, without the addition of drugs, is in itself beneficial and will result in faster recovery from attacks of MS. Recovery will eventually prevail to the extent that recovery will occur in any given attack. There is no evidence that treatment of MS attacks with any available medication results in superior long-term results. In general, if an attack is minor, treatment does not provide any advantage and is better avoided. For example, if a person has decreased vision from 20/20 (normal) to 20/40 or even 20/60 in one eye, vision will return without treatment, often quite quickly. Apart from the cost, high-dose steroids certainly have potential side effects and would be best avoided in such an attack. In those rare patients who suffer a complete loss of vision in one or both eyes, high-dose steroids result in the recovery of usable vision in a greater proportion of patients.

80. What are the side effects of the drugs that are used for the treatment of MS attacks? Are cataracts a result of steroid use? Is osteoporosis a complication of MS?

Side effects are common with steroids, whether these drugs are administered by mouth or by IV. Several categories of important side effects are distinguished: alteration of mood, formation of cataracts, increased risk of infection, impaired wound healing, loss of calcium from bone, ischemic necrosis of bone, and muscle damage, to mention only the more commonly recognized problems.

Cataracts

Cataracts are a well-known complication of steroid use. The risk of cataracts is related to the total dose of steroid used but varies greatly from person to person. The type of cataract is unique to the use of steroids and is easily recognized by ophthalmologists. As with other cataracts, extraction with lens replacement is the only real treatment. There seems to be little or no risk associated with ACTH use in MS.

Weight Gain and Altered Body Habitus

Steroids and ACTH result in an increased appetite. Their use can result in tremendous weight gain, even as much as 70 pounds in a few days. There is also a redistribution of body fat that women, in particular, do not like. Fat is deposited over the face and upper part of the chest and neck, abdomen, and buttocks. As easy as it is to gain the weight, it is just as difficult to take it off. When caloric intake is managed (restricted), the deposition of fat over the upper back, abdomen, and buttocks is minimized, but not eliminated. The alteration of body image may be traumatic, particularly to women. **Acne** often accompanies the use of steroids and ACTH. It can be easily managed with use of low doses of tetracycline antibiotics.

Infection

The use of steroids is associated with an increased risk of infection of all types, including viral, bacterial, fungal, and parasitic disease. Although viral infections are usually mentioned as a risk with steroid administration, including a risk of progressive multifocal leukoencephalopathy (PML), these infections are relatively uncommon. **Shingles** (herpes zoster) and flares of **genital herpes** are probably the most common viral infections seen.

Compared with viral infections, bacterial infections are a more practical problem. The most commonly encountered bacterial infections complicating the use of steroids include flare-ups of bladder and kidney infections (**cystitis** and **pyelonephritis**, respectively). Less commonly, skin wounds, pneumonias, and rarer infections can be problematic.

Although yeast infestation of throat (**thrush**) and **yeast vaginitis** are relatively common problems with steroid

Acne

A skin condition common in young people that is characterized by increased secretion from oil glands in the skin, accompanied by formation of comedones (blackheads).

Shingles

Skin infection caused by the herpes zoster virus. It is typically associated with pain.

Genital herpes

A contagious viral infection primarily affecting the genitals of men and women. It is characterized by recurrent clusters of vesicles and lesions in the affected areas and is caused by the herpes simplex-2 virus (HSV-2).

Cystitis

Inflammation of the bladder associated with symptoms of urinary frequency and urgency.

Pyelonephritis

An acute infection of the kidney associated with fever; it is contrasted with cystitis (a bladder infection), where fever does not occur.

treatment, they are usually easy to manage. **Systemic infections** are rare, but can occasionally be very serious. Fungal infections are unusual except accompanying chronic steroid use.

Parasitic infections such as **toxoplasmosis** and *pneumocystis* infection, which complicate HIV infection, are not common with steroid therapy. Nevertheless, they may occur with chronic steroid use, particularly if the steroids are used in combination with drugs such as Imuran and methotrexate.

Wound Healing

Surgical and other wounds heal more slowly in patients on steroids and are more likely to become infected. For those persons with bed sores, steroids are particularly problematic. Management of these patients should avoid even short-term steroids.

Bone Damage

The use of steroids results in the loss of calcium from bones, a phenomenon that underlies the development of **osteopenia** and osteoporosis. Subsequently, these conditions may lead to collapse of vertebrae and an increased risk of fracture of the long bones. An even more serious possibility is the increased likelihood of ischemic (aseptic) necrosis of the hips and other joints. We have found an especially high incidence of unrecognized aseptic necrosis in children treated with high-dose IV steroids prior to referral to our center. When this problem is diagnosed early, treatment can reverse or limit the amount of permanent joint damage. Conversely, advanced joint damage leaves only joint replacement as an option. Physicians and patients have to be aware of such potential complications. Difficulty in walking or pain in the knee may actually

---

Thrush

Throat infection by the yeast *Candida albicans*. It is a common complication with treatment consisting of antibiotics and steroids.

Yeast vaginitis

A common infection due to the yeast *Candida albicans*.

Surgical and other wounds heal more slowly in patients on steroids and are more likely to become infected.

Systemic infections

Any infection that causes generalized symptoms (as opposed to a localized infection). It is usually associated with a fever.

Toxoplasmosis

Infestation of the human body by the one-celled organism *Toxoplasma gondii*.

Pneumocystis

A one-celled organism that causes rapidly fatal lung infestations in AIDS patients.

Treatment of Multiple Sclerosis

indicate damage to a hip rather than a knee. In my long experience, I have never seen this complication in ACTH-treated patients.

Muscle Damage

Steroid therapy by any route, but especially with high- dose IV administration, weakens muscles. High-dose IV therapy carries with it the risk of severe muscle weakness, which, fortunately, is usually reversible. This complication is not seen with ACTH.

81. Why do I "go crazy" with steroids?

In most patients, there is an initial feeling of well- being induced by steroids, particularly when they are taken at lower doses. This mood elevation often is replaced by irritability with continued administration of steroids, particularly at higher doses. Psychotic behav- ior may follow simple mood elevation. Frank **manic psy- chosis** occurs in a small proportion of patients treated with steroids by any route of administration. Mood elevation can be managed using lithium carbonate and diazepam. Although it is not common, some patients may become depressed when they take steroids. ACTH use may occasionally be associated with these mood changes as well.

82. How do the side effects of ACTH and steroids compare?

The side effects of ACTH are generally similar to those of steroids taken orally or by IV administration, but are less severe. All of the side effects seen with steroids, including psychosis and bone injury, but not muscle weakness, may occur with ACTH. Certain hormones whose production is induced by ACTH and that are manufactured by the adrenal glands, known as "keto- steroids" (such as **testosterone**), have an anabolic (protein building) effect. As in athletes, the anabolic steroids that are induced by ACTH treatment are capable of making muscles somewhat stronger. In contrast, the net effect of steroids is catabolic (protein destroying).

Karen's comment:

When I was first diagnosed with MS, my doctor at the time prescribed steroids—specifically, oral prednisone, intravenous steroid methylprednisolone, and then more oral prednisone. As a result, I was simultaneously dealing with the diagnosis, having my body go through things it had never done before (such as vision loss, MRI [magnetic resonance imaging], and spinal tap), managing the logistics of a nurse for the IV steroids, processing the mounds of insurance forms, and coping with the side effects of the steroids.

Fortunately, I have low blood pressure, am not overweight, and manage my diet well, so I missed many of the side effects—but not all. I got the tell-tale "Cabbage Patch Doll" face such that my eyeglasses would barely squeeze on. For several months, I was "hyper" and unable to sleep from midnight to 4 A.M. I would alphabetically arrange our 1,000 books. Other odd things happened, such as when the hair on my arms fell out.

*Coming off the steroids was hard as well. My body was addicted. One day I yelled at my husband for eating a potato chip too loudly when he was three rooms away. On another day, I felt a loss of **adrenaline** and ate an entire box of Dots candy I grabbed from the shelf of our grocery store. All told, from first dose to last weaning pill, I had 6 months of steroids—2 months of intended benefit and 4 months for withdrawal. Almost 13 years later, I still have residual effects from that one event with steroids: I have some change in my body shape that is referred to as trunk effect, osteoporosis, and pre-cataract fibers in my eyes.*

Treatment of Multiple Sclerosis

Adrenaline
The principal hormone secreted by the adrenal medulla. This hormone is made from the amino acid tyrosine and is not a steroid. It makes the heart beat more forcefully and faster and raises the blood pressure. Adrenaline secretion is also part of the "fight-or-flight" response to stress.

83. I don't want steroids. Are other treatments available for MS attacks?

Traditionally, the management of MS centered on the use of extended periods of physical (and mental) rest, as it did for patients with tuberculosis or rheumatoid arthritis. Today, relapse management in MS seems to revolve around the use of steroids. ACTH was approved for the treatment of attacks of MS by the FDA in 1978 and remains the only drug approved for treatment of MS attacks. The IV form of ACTH is in very short supply, but the intramuscular form (Acthar Gel) is again in production and can be obtained with a prescription. Although it may be administered on an outpatient basis, careful medical monitoring is an absolute requirement. The drug has become very expensive, for reasons that are unclear, and insurance coverage is sometimes a problem.

84. Why are IV steroids given for attacks of MS?

Myelograms

X-ray studies of the spinal cord and spinal canal performed by the injection of contrast media. Computerized tomography and magnetic resonance imaging studies have largely replaced this procedure.

More than 30 years ago, after performing **myelograms** to rule out tumors, we found that the spinal cord was swollen during severe attacks of MS, causing paralysis. When CT scans of the brain and orbits became available to study patients with severe attacks of optic neuritis in 1972, we also found the optic nerves to be markedly swollen. We reasoned that with high doses of steroids we should be able to reduce the swelling in the spinal cord and optic nerve to prevent further damage from the lack of circulation in the affected areas of the nervous system. High-dose steroids did seem to work, often more quickly than with ACTH. However, many more side effects were found in patients with the use of high-dose steroids than with ACTH, which somewhat dissuaded us from using this form of treatment.

Many neurologists favor the use of steroids as being convenient, disregarding the lack of adequate controlled trials in MS.

The optic neuritis trial of IV methylprednisolone (Medrol) appeared to validate the use of a high dose (1 gram per day) as effective in speeding recovery from optic neuritis. Oral steroids, in contrast, did not accelerate recovery; and indeed, their use resulted in a relapse rate that was twice as high in that trial *for optic neuritis alone.* Although many neurologists have rationalized their prescription of oral steroids because of fatigue reduction and often restoration of a sense of well-being, they ignore a potentially higher posttreatment relapse rate. Oral steroids have not been demonstrated in any adequate trial to be useful treatment for optic neuritis or other MS relapses.

85. Are there treatments to prevent attacks and lessen risk of disability?

A variety of treatments are available to prevent attacks and reduce the risk of disability with MS—and the list of options is about to get longer. Three forms of interferon-beta and glatiramer acetate constitute the "ABC" first wave of injectable drug products. These drugs were modestly effective. Natalizumab (Tysabri), an intravenous drug, appears to be about twice as effective as the first-wave drugs. The first entries in a third wave of MS drugs, which include a number of oral products, are anticipated soon but are not yet available in the market. Two of these drugs—cladribine and fingolimod—have been reported to have effectiveness approaching that of Tysabri. Applications for their approval have been submitted to the FDA in the United States, with similar submissions being made to the appropriate regulatory agencies in Europe and Canada. Other oral products and two intravenous drugs are currently under investigation.

Successful clinical and MRI study results for three drugs, the so-called ABC (Avonex, Betaseron, Copaxone) drugs, resulted in FDA approval of these agents for the treatment of relapsing MS. The first to be approved was interferon-beta-1b (Betaseron, 1993), followed by interferon-beta-1a (Avonex, 1996, and Rebif, 2002), and glatiramer acetate (Copaxone, 1997). There is a marked reduction in new MRI lesions within the first month with the higher-dose interferon product Betaseron and, by inference, with Rebif. Unfortunately, none of these drugs is associated with any reduction of relapse rates within 6 months of initiation of treatment. After 2 years of treatment, exacerbations are reduced by approximately 30% for each of these approved products. Although subcutaneous interferon-beta-1b (Betaseron) and interferon-beta-1a (Rebif) have similar salutary reductions in exacerbations at 1 year, this effect is not seen in this time frame with either Avonex or Copaxone. Separate head-to-head studies comparing Rebif and Betaseron with Copaxone have shown no differences in clinical benefits achieved with Copaxone in 2-year trials.

The higher-dose interferons have more side effects associated with them with their initial use. Both high-dose forms of interferon-beta are associated with injection site reactions as well as significant "flu-like" reactions, principally consisting of fever, headache, and diffuse aches and pains. The introduction of an escalating dosage schedule has markedly reduced the severity of these systemic reactions. Local skin reactions may be prominent, although these side effects become less severe and may disappear within a few weeks of initiating therapy.

Similarly, glatiramer acetate is associated with injection site reactions, albeit half as frequently (about 40%) as with the higher-dose interferons, and an anxiety-like syndrome with chest tightness in a smaller proportion of patients. A flu-like syndrome is relatively uncommon in glatiramer-treated patients. Severe skin reactions appear to occur about as frequently as with high-dose interferons. Allergic manifestations, including anaphylactic-like reactions, are also seen with this drug.

Natalizumab (Tysabri)

The clinical outcomes in the Phase 3 trials of natalizumab (Tysabri) showed benefits that greatly surpassed those of the products previously on the market. Natalizumab reduced the risk of sustained disability for 3 months by 42% and for 6 months by 54%. This latter standard was used to describe the reductions achieved with Avonex and Rebif. In MRI studies, a similar early reduction in **gadolinium**-enhancing lesions was seen with high-dose interferon-beta as well as with natalizumab.

The AFFIRM (natalizumab safety and efficacy in relapsing–remitting MS) study was a 2-year, multicenter, randomized, placebo-controlled investigation of a fixed intravenous 300-mg dose of natalizumab administered every 4 weeks. Of the total enrollment of 942 patients, 627 patients received active treatment. On the basis of the primary outcome for the first year—namely, a 66% reduction of relapses and a favorable safety and tolerance profile—the FDA approved the drug for the prevention of relapses in November 2004. The primary outcome measure for the completed 2-year study was the impact of treatment on the prevention of sustained disability (defined as a 3-month

Treatment of Multiple Sclerosis

Gadolinium

An injected contrast material used to make blood vessels (or tumors) more visible on MRI brain or other tissue scans.

increase in disability by one point on the EDSS). The reduction of relapses was sustained through the second year, with a 42% reduction in sustained disability. Using the same criteria employed in the Avonex trial (sustained disability by one point on the EDSS for 6 months); a 54% reduction was reported.

The SENTINEL (safety and efficacy of natalizumab in combination with Avonex [interferon-beta-1a]) study was a second ongoing 2-year randomized multicenter, placebo-controlled, double-blind study of 1,171 patients with relapsing–remitting MS. The same dose of natalizumab (300 mg IV every 4 weeks) was used. In this trial, patients who had been treated with Avonex (interferon-beta-1a) but who had experienced one or more relapses while on treatment were randomized to receive natalizumab or placebo on a 1:1 basis. Avonex was continued throughout the study for both groups. The Avonex group consisted of 582 patients, and the combined treatment group had 589 patients. The outcome measures for this second 2-year study were the same as those for the AFFIRM study. Natalizumab reduced the frequency of relapse by 54% versus placebo.

Karen's comment:

I took natalizumab in December 1997 as part of a Phase 2 trial for what was then called Antegren. In October 1997, I was feeling great. My MS was seemingly nonexistent. I was in New Jersey enjoying the fall leaves, biking, and picking raspberries; I even thought about trying to teach in the spring term. I did not realize that I was pregnant and soon to miscarry.

After the miscarriage, we called Dr. Sheremata, who asked when I was next going to be in Miami. I told him in a week, for my father's 65th birthday. He warned us that it was likely that I would have a flare-up. As I enjoyed a long weekend in Florida, I felt a bit smug and a lot relieved that I had not had a flare-up and almost canceled my appointment with Dr. Sheremata for that Tuesday. On Monday night, I was tired but still okay. By Tuesday morning, I could not see out of my right eye, and neither of my legs worked very well.

My father and I went to see Dr. Sheremata; we discussed ACTH, and Dr. Sheremata mentioned a drug trial. The Phase 2 study was designed for patients who were within 48 hours of the beginning of a flare-up, and I was certainly in that group. I had to agree to be studied for 3 months at regular intervals, including MRIs, physical exams, and blood work. Adding insult to injury, I had to take a pregnancy test to make sure that I was not pregnant. The informed consent agreement was standard, but what I had seen as sensible as a practicing lawyer seemed ridiculous as a patient in the midst of a flare-up: Ill and with poor vision, how informed could I be about an experiment for something only a few humans had tried? The prior trial for a different MS drug had been halted when patients had what the FDA termed "strong negative events" (i.e., heart attacks).

I called my husband in New Jersey, who—just as when I was first diagnosed with MS—was worried and had difficulty imagining how I could be so ill because 2 days ago, when he had last seen me, I was fine. I felt a bit like the castaways on Gilligan's Island. I had left for a 3-day weekend, only to be gone for 3 months as a guinea pig.

How did we decide to do the trial? Dr. Sheremata gave us caring, intelligent, and neutral information. We prayed. And we went forward.

The next day, another patient and I had infusions of drug or placebo. Over many hours, Dr. Sheremata observed us and told us about the Macintosh apples of his childhood. My father nervously ate the sandwiches, as the other patient and I were too tense to eat, and my husband called regularly. As we left the hospital and went over the bridge to the island where we live, I thought about what I had done; I wondered if my hair had turned purple. I wondered what was happening in my body. I could not undo it. The next day I felt great. The independent doctor who was doing the physical exams said I either got drug or had great prayer and placebo. During my exam before I had the IV, he had told me that I needed a foot brace and a walker. Now I was biking 10 miles. It turned out that I received the drug and not placebo, and as always, I had great prayer.

Despite the marked salutary effect on relapses, the fact that the full impact of the drug on relapses was realized by 6 weeks of treatment, and the accompanying reduction of sustained disability, Tysabri was withdrawn from the market shortly after its approval by the FDA. Two of the 589 patients who had received Avonex and Tysabri (one for 23 months and the other for 37 months) developed progressive multifocal leukoencephalopathy (PML), a serious brain infection caused by the JC virus. In addition, a patient with Crohn's disease who had received multiple drug therapies developed this disease. Of the approximately 3,000 patients with MS, Crohn's disease, or rheumatoid arthritis, the only patients who developed PML were those two MS patients on combined Tysabri and Avonex therapy and the patient with Crohn's disease who had received multiple immunosuppressants as well as Tysabri.

After a full review of the facts by an FDA panel, Tysabri was returned to the market coupled with a comprehensive risk management program, the TOUCH (Tysabri Outreach: Unified Commitment to Health) Program, in May 2006. It was concluded that the risk of PML was about 1 per 1000. In the United States, Tysabri has been used primarily for treatment failure, as judged by the treating neurologist, with a requirement for close management consisting of clinical examination and brain MRI monitoring.

As of January 12, 2010, there had been 31 new cases of PML among a total of more than 60,000 Tysabri-treated patients. The risk of this infection is 0.47 per 1000 for the patients in the original studies who have since continued on Tysabri—lower than the risk calculated from the trials that led to approval. This is a relatively smaller group, so final conclusions must be guarded. It also appears that the risk for PML may increase over a period of time, a trend that had been anticipated. The risk appears to be higher in Europe, where a PML risk management program was not implemented, than in the United States, where the monitoring program is mandatory. From observations in Europe, it appears that prior treatment with methotrexate or mitoxantrone (Novantrone), both of which are potent immunosuppressants, may increase that risk. Despite the 20 to 30% incidence of viremia with the JC virus induced by steroid usage, infection with this virus is extremely rare in conjunction with Tysabri, making JC virus testing monitoring appear unhelpful.

Withdrawal of Tysabri coupled with plasma exchange has resulted in survival of the majority, but not all, of the patients who developed PML. However, a major MS attack inevitably follows such cessation of treatment. These severe attacks resemble the immune reconstitution syndrome that occurs in AIDS patients with PML who are managed with optimized antiviral therapy.

Treatment of Multiple Sclerosis

New patients considered for Tysabri treatment include those who have not responded to standard treatment and patients who require aggressive immunosuppression to stabilize their illness.

New patients considered for Tysabri treatment include those who have not responded to standard treatment and patients who require aggressive immunosuppression to stabilize their illness. They must be off steroids and standard treatments and counseled about the risk of PML prior to enrollment in the TOUCH program.

Karen's comment:

On November 23, 2004, 7 years after my first infusion of natalizumab as part of the drug trial, Tysabri was approved by the FDA. The next day our local pharmacist ordered a vial for me. There were few infusion centers open right away and my MS was worsening. Dr. Goodman (my general practitioner/endocrinologist/gynecologist) volunteered to give me my infusion. He reasoned that he had given IVs as a resident and that not much about the process had changed in the 40 years since. He was surprised that we were concerned that this could be a burden for him, noting that treating patients with effective medicine is what doctors are supposed to do. So on December 21, 2004, I took the vial of Tysabri to Dr. Goodman in our Playmate cooler and had my first "commercial" infusion.

Although Dr. Goodman offered to give me this one infusion, he is still giving them to me today. Not only does he give us his time and skill, but the entire office staff is involved. Rachel, one of the nurses, handles all the interactions with Biogen. She has been known to thicken her native Scottish brogue when she feels it will accomplish something to help a patient. Other staff help with the insurance labyrinth, scheduling, drawing blood, and tending to my father, including slipping him as many as six chocolates during one infusion.

At first, my infusions were medically perfect but nevertheless a bit rudimentary, beginning with finding a coat hanger to hang the intravenous solution bag on. Now years later, I have graduated to having my own IV pole. My father and I have a routine we began in the early days of Tysabri and continue to this day as to what to bring to each infusion: a craft I make for each staff member in their respective favorite color; a snack for during the infusion; a folder with all my blood test results; spare latex-free Snoopy band aids; a sparkly purple glove to keep the hand of my infusion arm warm; and the menu for the local deli so we can order Reuben sandwiches for the trip home.

As part of Tysabri's return to the market in 2006, Biogen, along with the FDA, developed a program called TOUCH (Tysabri Outreach: Unified Commitment to Health). This program carefully monitors all aspects of Tysabri, including the prescribing doctors, the infusing locations, the distribution, and the patients who receive it. There are strict guidelines and requirements for each under the program. For each infusion there is an administrative process, but for the patient it is fairly straightforward: Once you have a prescription from your neurologist, then the infusion location does the rest.

Most MS patients do not tolerate warm temperatures; I am in the small group who do not handle cold temperatures well. Understandably, places that give infusions tend to be cold for the comfort of the majority of patients, and I have to prepare for this. On the day of the infusion, I have a kindly massage therapist come to work on the arm being infused to make sure it does not spasm due to the cold and immobility during the 2-hour infusion time. Once I am at the infusion site, the appointment starts with a general physical exam. Next a series of questions must be read aloud to the patient concerning other medications and possible changes since the last infusion. Then the infusion begins. The Tysabri is administered intravenously for approximately 1 hour and is followed by a saline solution. Then I go home, eat my cholesterol-rich, artery-clogging Reuben sandwich, rest a bit, feel much better, and do the same thing 4 weeks later.

When I am "home south" in Florida, I continue to get my infusions with Dr. Goodman; when I am "home north" in New Jersey, I have infusions at an oncologist's office in New York City. There are no chocolates but I get great medical care from Dr. Gattani. Her office manager, Pavan, uses his calming Indian accent to smoothly negotiate the TOUCH process with Biogen. Unlike at Dr. Goodman's office, where the other patients are generally healthy and I am the least functioning, at Dr. Gattani's office, the other patients are getting chemotherapy for cancers. It is a good perspective setter. One day last year, when I was feeling particularly sorry for myself and useless, in frustration I thought, "All I am good for is growing hair." When I got a grip on myself, I thought of the chemotherapy patients and was reminded that growing hair is not something to take for granted and that I could do for others. Ten inches of hair later, I was able to donate my ponytail to benefit people who have lost their hair.

86. Is there a treatment that stops MS?

As noted in previous questions, several treatments have now been proven, in a series of trials, to reduce the risk of relapses in MS. The most recently approved drug, Tysabri, has the greatest benefit in this regard, leading to a 66% reduction in relapses. Although in their respective trials most of the drugs have been shown to decrease the risk of progression, it is not correct to say that they are capable of "stopping MS." The benefits of Betaseron, Avonex, Rebif, and Tysabri appear somewhat similar in this regard. Some MS patients have milder illness than others, and aggressive management, with the consequent more prominent side effects, may not be indicated.

Some evidence suggests that Novantrone, the most aggressive treatment approved, stabilizes the majority of progressive, or worsening, MS patients. Although it may be tempting to use this more aggressive treatment in patients with relapsing–remitting MS, as has been done in Europe, important side effects from this drug must be considered. Although all forms of treatment for MS (and virtually all medications) have side effects, the specific issues associated with Novantrone, such as the risk of leukemia (rare) and cardiac complications, cannot be ignored.

Karen's comment:

Tysabri comes close to stopping my MS. As with any drug, there were many obstacles and checkpoints before it got to market. Natalizumab seems to have had one of the longer and more roller-coaster-like routes to market and beyond. During the 7 years between my first and second infusions, I went through as many changes as the corporations that owned the drug, the FDA, and then some. I had more than 15 flare-ups, tried (without benefit) an interferon, volunteered for several drug trials that did not materialize, spent more than a year at a 5.5 disability level [on the EDSS], lost function in several areas, and considered chemotherapy.

After the second infusion, I slept for 3 days and woke up stronger and stayed stronger than I had been for many years. There were no negative side effects. I felt like I was going to get a chance to get better. I had been having flare-ups every few months and felt like Sisyphus—each time I would get even a foothold, I would get rolled back down the mountain of MS. Two infusions later, the drug was withdrawn from the market.

In February 2005, when Tysabri was voluntarily removed from the market, I was more scared and upset than the day I was diagnosed. Perhaps that was because I had a greater understanding of the implications; perhaps it was because I had begun to think I would regain my old me. I was in the process of updating my resume with thoughts of soon returning to teaching legal ethics. My husband saw the news via an alert he had on his computer for information about Tysabri and called me. A few minutes later, he called me again to tell me that he had used some of our savings to purchase six vials of the drug from a pharmacy. I told him that there was no chance I would take a medicine that had been removed from the market, albeit voluntarily, because there had to be a reason for the removal.

I was wrong. For 8 months (we extended the interval between each infusion to make it last), I continued to take Tysabri. Each month we intentionally examined whether I should have the infusion, each month I decided to have the infusion, and each month I had it and grew stronger. As the number of vials in our refrigerator dwindled, I tried to enjoy the well days. And then we ran out. In December I had a major relapse from which I still have not fully recovered.

After Tysabri was approved to return to the market, I began my infusions again. Although I am demonstrably better than I would be without it, I have not (yet?) returned to where I was before it was withdrawn. I will stay on it as long as Dr. Sheremata, the FDA, and my body permit. As I said to the FDA advisory committee on March 6, 2006, "Off Tysabri, on a good day I am a 5.5 on the EDSS scale, on lots of coffee, facing chemotherapy. On Tysabri, it is an even better day; I am a 1.5 on the EDSS scale, on my bike, facing the road ahead."

87. Would starting the ABC drugs prevent progression of MS? Will it really make a difference?

Yes! The so-called ABC drugs (Avonex, Betaseron, Copaxone), plus Rebif have been proven to reduce the risk of attacks in relapsing forms of MS. The original interferon-beta-1b (Betaseron) studies reported in 1993 (leading to approval later that year) were not designed to show a reduction in the risk of disability. The subsequent interferon-beta-1a (Avonex and Rebif) studies were designed to detect the effectiveness of treatment in preventing "sustained" disability as well as the impact on relapse rates. More recently, the benefit of Betaseron in reducing the risk of progression in secondary progressive disease has been established. Proving this effect was a more difficult task, as no evidence of this benefit was found in studies of other interferon-beta products. Interestingly, the reduction in the risk of progression noted in the Betaseron studies was evident only in patients who continued to relapse as well as exhibit progression of their illness between attacks (which defines secondary progressive MS).

Using drugs does make a difference in MS. Studies have proven that the interferon-beta products (Avonex, Betaseron, and Rebif) approved for use in MS have a benefit not only in reducing the risk of attacks, but also in reducing the risk of "sustained" disability (progression), although it is not realized in everyone who takes these drugs. Importantly, the benefit of all of these drugs has been shown to be better when they are instituted with the first attack of neurological disease—that is, at the very onset of clinical MS. In addition, newly reported

The so-called ABC drugs (Avonex, Betaseron, Copaxone), plus Rebif have been proven to reduce the risk of attacks in relapsing forms of MS.

evidence has shown that in half of all patients who are treated with interferon-beta, certain genes are turned on and attacks of MS seem to be completely prevented. Obviously, longer-term, more extensive studies will be needed to confirm this finding, but it is certainly very exciting news. These pharmacogenetics studies are being performed in virtually all new drug studies.

The pivotal studies of Copaxone did not show any impact on prevention of disability. In contrast, a 6-year, longitudinal follow-up study of a portion of the original study participants was interpreted to show an impressive prevention of disability in approximately two-thirds of those followed. More recent head to head studies of Copaxone with interferon-beta-1a (Rebif) and interferon-beta-1b (Betaseron) have now shown clinical similar outcomes for Copaxone and the interferon products. However, as previously observed, accumulation of new brain lesions continued with Copaxone but not the interferon products.

There is no test that can predict therapeutic success. Nevertheless, repeated examinations by experienced neurologists and MRI scans can provide information about how an individual patient is responding to treatment. Generally, apart from examinations and MRI scans, if you feel well, you probably are okay.

88. How do these drugs compare?

In addition to the two comparative drug studies in MS mentioned in Question 87, the EVIDENCE trial compared low-dose interferon-beta-1a (Avonex, 30 micrograms, once weekly) to high-dose interferon-beta-1a (Rebif, 44 micrograms, three times weekly). This comparison was conducted in the form of a single-blind design study. Superior results at 6, 12, and 16 months were seen in those patients taking the higher dose (Rebif). Interestingly, the data from the earlier pivotal studies of both drugs showed similar outcomes in patients completing 2 years of therapy, as the investigators reported. For the published trial results, it would appear that in the short-term, at least, early institution of high-dose (44 micrograms, three times weekly) interferon-beta-1a is more efficacious than low-dose interferon-beta-1a (30 micrograms, once weekly). It also has to be pointed out that the regimen of 22 micrograms given three times weekly (66 micrograms weekly) produced results that were reported to be inferior to those obtained with 44 micrograms given three times weekly in the pivotal Rebif study.

89. How do the (FDA-approved) drugs used in MS prevent attacks?

Interferon-alpha and interferon-beta-1b were first used in MS studies because of their known antiviral properties. As yet, there is no accepted evidence proving that either acute or chronic viral infection has any direct role in the causation of MS attacks or in the progression of this disease. There have been numerous studies of what the interferons do in the human body and, specifically, how they affect the mechanisms of tissue damage that occur in conjunction with MS. Both interferons produce a number of effects in the body that should have benefits in MS.

Among their other properties, interferons decrease the activation (turning on) of lymphocytes and macrophages in a number of different ways. In addition, they decrease the ability of activated cells to stick to the inside of the blood vessels of the brain and spinal cord via adhesion molecules. The interferons also interfere with cells already stuck to the inside of the blood vessels and hinder their

Matrix metalloprotease (MMP)

Any member of a group of secreted neutral proteases that degrade the collagens of the extracellular matrix. Members of this group are important in the integrity of the blood–brain barrier. MMP9 appears to be the most important of the group in this regard; it is inhibited by interferon-beta (Avonex, Betaseron, and Rebif).

ability to initiate the series of events that allow the cells to eat a hole through the blood vessel's wall. This is accomplished through a number of mechanisms, including the inhibition of **matrix metalloproteases (MMP)**. It is generally accepted that these mechanisms are important in conferring the benefits of Betaseron, Avonex, and Rebif in MS.

Glatiramer acetate (Copaxone), although not an interferon, appears to function as a decoy for the immune system. It prevents myelin-like proteins from activating mechanisms that might otherwise cause additional myelin damage. Extrapolating from animal studies, there appear to be a number of beneficial effects on immune function from the use of this drug. Recent evidence suggests that Copaxone plays an important role in MS by switching off cytotoxic lymphocytes (CD8+ cells) and turning on immunosuppressive activity.

90. Why aren't drugs used together in MS treatment to get a better effect?

In a form of shorthand that immunologists use, helper T-cell immune function is referred to as "CD4 Th1 function," and suppressor inducer T-cell (immunoregulatory) function is referred to as a type of "CD4 Th2 function." The net result with both the interferons and glatiramer acetate is to shift immune function away from Th1 activity and toward Th2 function. It would seem, at least theoretically, that combinations of these drugs might be more effective in altering immune function to increase CD4 Th2 function. To this end, a continuing pivotal study funded by the National Institutes of Health, known as the CombiRx study, is exploring the potential benefit of interferon-beta-1a (Avonex) versus glatiramer acetate (Copaxone) versus the combination of these drugs. A pharmacogenetics study is coupled with this study, as with all of the more modern studies. Ideally, the findings from these studies will help predict who will respond best to which drug, or which drug combination.

91. What is Tysabri, and why was this drug temporarily withdrawn from the market?

Natalizumab (Tysabri) is a monoclonal antibody to an adhesion molecule (VLA-4) that was approved by the FDA for use in MS patients in November 2004, on the basis of studies that showed good results for the drug— namely, a marked (66%) reduction in MS exacerbations, a 91% reduction in gadolinium-enhancing brain lesions (per MRI study), and a good safety and tolerance profile. This reduced exacerbation rate was sustained through the entire 2 years of the clinical trials studying the drug. In addition, these effects were accompanied by an impressive 42% reduction in the risk of sustained progression of disability over the 2 years of the study. The reduction in the risk of attacks was achieved by selectively blocking one (and only one) Velcro-like molecule on lymphocytes, thereby preventing these cells from attaching to the inside of brain and spinal cord (cerebral) blood vessels. Extrapolating from animal studies, this action effectively prevented the lymphocytic cells from crossing the blood–brain barrier. The dramatically superior effectiveness of Tysabri in preventing attacks of MS, which was also seen after 2 years of therapy, confirmed the importance of blood lymphocytes' and macrophages' role in attacks of MS, and also proved that this step (attachment via a specific adhesion molecule VLA-4) is a central factor in attacks of MS.

Three cases of PML in study participants (two patients with MS and one patient with Crohn's disease) were recognized just as the drug was put on the U.S. market, prompting a voluntary withdrawal of Tysabri by its manufacturer. The risk of developing PML with Tysabri use was determined to be 1:1000. Eventually, the drug was reintroduced in tandem with a risk management program (TOUCH) directed at monitoring patients for PML. No use of steroids and approved treatments for MS within 3 weeks of starting Tysabri is required to begin taking Tysabri, and patients must participate in an ongoing clinical monitoring program. Use of the drug in the United States is essentially limited to patients who have not responded to standard treatment. The manufacturer controls all drug shipments and monitors compliance with the rules.

New cases of PML have occurred since the reintroduction of Tysabri, with the majority of these cases occurring in Europe, where the risk management program was not required. Nevertheless, the risk of PML is not higher than originally reported. The use of Tysabri in Europe is under review by the European regulatory agency at the present time.

Karen's comment:

For me, the question is how Tysabri returned to the market. I get cranky when I think of its removal. From the day it was withdrawn, my husband, my father, and countless others independently and collectively began a campaign to try to bring the drug back to the market. We felt that we were uniquely positioned to know or have access to many people who could help in significant ways and that we had the responsibility to use this power for something we hoped would benefit all MS patients. As time went on and my condition deteriorated, we were not sure I would be able to take Tysabri again even if it came back on the market, and prepared for me to start chemotherapy instead. Yet we felt it was important to keep trying—if not for me, then for all MS patients to have the right to choose to take Tysabri.

My husband relentlessly raised the issue of Tysabri with anyone he met. Friends, family, colleagues—all contacted someone who, in turn, contacted someone else. And so it went. Eventually we had amassed a network of both regular citizens and powerful people to help. The people who were part of this effort included shareholders in the pharmaceutical companies that developed and manufactured Tysabri, MS patients, academics, clergy, friends, family, business executives, doctors, regulators, economists, and biologists. People wanted to help, for which we are eternally grateful. Through this network we were able to have more than 1000 people write the FDA, the pharmaceutical companies, and legislators about Tysabri.

A year after the drug was withdrawn, the FDA scheduled hearings to help determine whether and under what conditions to put Tysabri back on the market. So many people wanted to testify (not all in support of Tysabri's return) that the hearings were held in a ballroom of a large hotel. More than 400 people from the public and the press attended. Several interest groups and 40 individuals were scheduled to testify. Each person was assigned a number and an order to speak and allotted 5 minutes to speak. Next to each microphone there was a timer clock: At the $4\frac{1}{2}$-minute mark, a yellow light came on; at 5 minutes, the microphone automatically shut off. It was emotional to listen to people who traveled long distances at their own expense to plead and pour their hearts out, while also trying to manage their MS symptoms. Often they were unable to finish their statements in the allotted time, which made it all the more poignant. I can still hear the voice of the woman who brought a photo of her son to place next to her at the podium and only managed to say the word "please" *before she ran out of time. In some respects, perhaps it was all she really needed to say.*

My father, my husband, and I testified. I was unable to sit up for very long and so was lying on the floor of the ballroom until just before our turn. One of the individuals who were "angels unaware" came over to meet us and sat next to me on the floor. Her name was Bonnie—she was the daughter of my sister's friend's mother's bridge partner and she was there to cheer us on. She brought us cookies and a hug. We later learned she was also with the FDA, in the area of clinical trial patient's rights, and she herself was suffering with—and has since passed away from—a terminal illness. David and I were termed a "group" and given 6 minutes together but were able to have our say with 0.09 second to spare. A link to our testimony is http:// www.youtube.com/watch?v=MHFJuEsHurI. We have been told that our statements were instrumental in the positive outcome of the hearings. I would not have been able to testify without the training I had as a lawyer and professor, prayer, and the hug from Bonnie.

The FDA committee unanimously voted to recommend to the FDA to return natalizumab to the market—only the second time a prescription drug has been returned to the market after having been withdrawn. Since the return of Tysabri to the market, we hear almost daily from people who are on the medication. One person wrote us that she previously was unable to walk and now she was able to dance at her daughter's wedding; another person took a vacation with his wife for the first time in 20 years; and one person regained her vision and was able to drive her child to daycare. Words like "hope," "future," "relief," "confidence," "strength," "joy," and "wow" are repeated in note after note that we receive.

To answer the question I posed: How did Tysabri return to the market?

Tysabri returned to the market because many people who have MS, and many who do not, worked together and created a change for the good.

92. What are the side effects of the drugs that are used to prevent attacks? Why should I take drugs that have side effects? How do the side effects compare?

The approved drugs reduce the risk of exacerbations as well as the risk of disability. They were approved by the FDA because of their safety as well as their effectiveness in treating MS. In reality, most recipients of the drugs available for MS treatment (Betaseron, Avonex, Rebif, and Copaxone) do experience side effects. Flu-like symptoms occur in the majority of patients early in interferon-beta therapy regardless of which one is chosen. Generally, they are more prominent with higher-dose interferon-beta (Betaseron and Rebif) and less noticeable with low-dose interferon-beta (Avonex) and for Copaxone. The higher-dose interferons, however, have a more rapid onset of benefit, as judged from MRI studies and the pivotal drug study results.

The approved drugs reduce the risk of exacerbations as well as the risk of disability.

Local reactions to injections under the skin (subcutaneous injections) are less frequent for Copaxone, about half as common as compared with injections of interferon-beta (Betaseron and Rebif). Localized redness of the skin decreases over time but almost always persists to some degree in the majority of patients. Most patients readily accept it as a nuisance. A few people will develop little dents in the skin in areas where the drug has been injected (lipodystrophy), similar to areas where insulin has been administered in patients with diabetes. Others will develop hard nodules under the skin at the injection site. Some patients who are given Avonex or

Rebif experience some stinging sensation with injections, which may be due to the acidity of the solution.

Copaxone, despite its requirement for daily injections, is associated with fewer side effects than the interferon-beta products, but the full benefit is delayed, as it is with Avonex. Copaxone induces a local reaction in approximately 40% of patients; half complain of some pain at the injection site. Again, this effect does not appear to be a major problem. A few patients develop prominent skin rashes. Approximately one-fourth of patients experience a transient feeling of anxiety or shortness of breath, which is ordinarily a minor issue, but occasionally is more severe and longer lasting.

In summary, the side effects from Betaseron and Rebif are initially more prominent but tend to subside sooner than those experienced by patients who are treated with Avonex. Generally, the side effects from Copaxone are less severe. For all of these products, there are considerable differences in side effects from one individual to another. The reason why certain patients tolerate one drug better than others remains unknown.

93. What is "the vaccine for MS?"

There continues to be a great deal of confusion in the minds of many MS patients and family members about a "vaccine for MS." Some seem to think of any injectable drug as a vaccine, but this is not a correct concept. All of the medications currently approved by the FDA for chronic (long-term) use in MS are drugs but are not vaccines, although their use is intended to prevent periods of ill health. Interferon-beta-1b (Betaseron), interferon-beta-1a (Avonex and Rebif), and glatiramer acetate (Copaxone®) are injectable drugs but are not vaccines.

A vaccine, which is ordinarily injected, stimulates the immune system, resulting in antibody formation to the injected protein or proteins or a direct effect of lymphocytes against those proteins or cells that have specific proteins on their surface. Several vaccines against cells in the immune system have been used in research trials. Despite early enthusiasm for this approach, no useful results have emerged from those studies. Such studies are to be distinguished from studies of altered proteins that attempt to induce immune tolerance; the latter studies are continuing.

94. Is there going to be a vaccine for MS?

There is ongoing research into T-cell vaccines for MS. The original experiments in Europe attracted a great deal of interest. They involved injecting crude preparations of blood lymphocytes into patients in an attempt to eliminate or reduce the number of "activated" lymphocytes in MS patients. Ongoing studies involve a more sophisticated selection of cells to be targeted for removal by immune action. They appear to be tolerable and effective to a degree, but they do not result in a long-lasting benefit. Other stalled studies have attempted to induce immune tolerance without provoking a direct attack on existing cells; only preliminary data on their safety have been published. No studies of this third-generation type of vaccine are currently under way.

95. What does alternative medicine have to offer?

There is no lack of "alternative" approaches to the holistic management of MS or for specific or individual problems. The vast majority of these "therapies" are of questionable value, whereas some are potentially dangerous. However, in the right hands, **hypnotism** and **biofeedback** may be very helpful approaches.

96. Is hypnotism helpful in MS?

The use of hypnotism is not to be taken lightly. Certainly, only trained professionals who are aware of MS and who are in communication with the patient's treating physicians should use hypnotism. There is no generally accepted use of this modality in MS, but there may be a place for hypnotism in combination with psychotherapy.

97. Is biofeedback useful in MS?

In recent years, biofeedback has become commonly used in the management of pain in pain clinics. The use of biofeedback now appears to be generally well accepted. Past studies with Dr. Ronald Melzack at McGill University revealed a surprise result, however, patients receiving workers' compensation because of back pain responded better to biofeedback than MS patients with back pain did. Despite this finding, biofeedback may prove helpful in some MS patients. More sophisticated approaches to biofeedback have recently evolved from spinal cord injury centers and other medical clinics.

98. Is there a cure for MS on the near horizon?

The old aphorism "Nothing is impossible; some things are just more difficult" is an appropriate response to this question. A cure for MS is not likely. Just as men and women recover from heart attacks and lead productive lives, so patients can function well with a diagnosis of MS.

Although a half-century ago rational treatment of MS seemed improbable, if not impossible, treatments proven to reduce the risk of attacks and disability have become a reality in the last two decades. Consequently, we all eagerly await new developments in the field of MS treatment. Better experimental treatment designs and more effective drugs are anticipated. If a drug is to be used, it must first be shown to be safe. Then, and only then, is it permissible to investigate the effectiveness of the new drug in patients.

Efficacy studies of natalizumab (Tysabri) appeared in the *New England Journal of Medicine* 6 years ago. It was reported to be the most effective drug studied for prevention of relapses in MS. On February 4, 2010, results of the first of the new oral agents (fingolimod and cladribine) from pivotal treatment trials were reported in the *New England Journal of Medicine*. These two drugs are reported to have effectiveness approaching that reported for Tysabri. The documented 1:1000 risk of PML with Tysabri suggests that, apart from other concerns regarding other infections and malignant disease (and macular edema for fingolimod, specifically), there may be a similar potential risk of PML with these agents. A risk management program, therefore, is expected to be instituted once these drugs reach the U.S. market.

Karen's comment:

One of my nieces was in an advanced science program at the age of 7 years. The class assignment was to invent something new; her invention was something to fix "multiple skleroys." Although her spelling was not accurate, her sentiment is one shared by many. When I was first diagnosed in 1996, the pundits predicted a cure for MS in 5 years. Five years later, the cure was anticipated within 10 years. Now it is said, "Perhaps within my lifetime."

Over the years, my thinking about cure has also evolved— not just about an ever-extending timeline, but also about

Treatment of Multiple Sclerosis

the meaning of cure. As a retired lawyer and nonretired bibliophile, the definition of a word is important to me. "Cure"—does it mean all people who get MS after a cure is found will be made disease-free; all people who have MS now will become disease-free or symptom-free; existing MS brain and nerve damage will be repaired; or no one will get MS?

Until a cure is found, whatever it means, I view my role as threefold: to give my support, financial and otherwise, to those people and organizations working on a cure; to volunteer my body, alive and dead, to researchers working on a cure; and to keep myself physically, mentally, and spiritually as strong as possible to be ready for a cure and to be ready if a cure is not found in my lifetime. I have confidence in my niece.

99. What is the future?

Studies of new molecules have continued to provide candidate therapies for MS. A third wave of drugs, orally administered, is emerging from recent drug trials and is likely to result in the introduction of new treatments for MS in the near future. Two new oral agents with unique mechanisms of action are being reviewed by the FDA in the United States and by comparable regulatory agencies in Europe. Another two or three drugs probably will also be submitted for approval in the next year or two. Oral cladribine and fingolimod are the first new drug applications being considered at the present time. **Figure 8** compares the mechanisms of actions of these drugs with that of Tysabri.

Oral *cladribine* was submitted for marketing approval by EMD Serono, based on large double-blind, placebo-controlled trials in MS. The drug was originally introduced about 20 years ago for the treatment of leukemia.

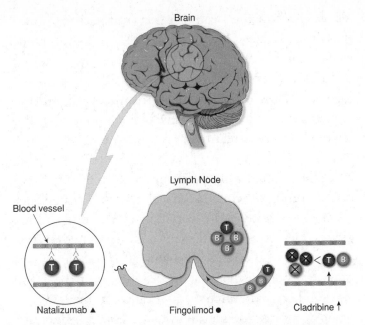

Figure 8   Comparison of Mode of Action of Three Drugs for MS—Tysabri (natalizumab), fingolimod, and cladribine. *Left*: Natalizumab (Tysabri) (△) attached to α4β1-Integrin, blocking attachment of activated [CD4+ & CD8+] lymphocytes to the receptor (VCAM) on the blood vessel wall in the brain and spinal cord. *Middle*: Fingolimod results in the lymphocyte receptor (●), required to exit lymph nodes anywhere in the body, becoming internalized in the cells. As a result, T-cells and B-cells can enter lymph nodes but cannot leave and enter blood stream. Note that there are no lymph nodes inside the brain and spinal cord. *Right*: Cladribine entering lymphocytes is not metabolized by the important enzyme *adenosine deaminase*. Instead it is broken down and forms molecules called deoxyribonucleotides which primarily damages T-cells. CD20 lymphocytes ("pre-pre B-cells") are also damaged but to a lesser extent.

Cladribine escapes a molecule called adenosine deaminase. Congenital deficiency of this enzyme results in severe combined immunodeficiency (SCID) in children. Cladribine avoids inactivation by the enzyme adenosine deaminase, thereby resulting in the production of toxic deoxyribonucleotides, molecules. The production of these molecules reduces T-lymphocyte subtypes (CD4 and CD8 **T cells** more than CD19, which are pre-B-cell populations) and produces immunosuppression. In the drug trials reported in February 2010,

T cell

A type of lymphocyte that develops in the thymus. "Killer T cell" is a term commonly used to describe a cytotoxic T cell. T cells are thymus-dependent lymphocytes that fail to develop in the absence of a functional thymus.

relapses in the active treatment trial arms in the 96 weeks study were reduced by 57.6% and 54.5%, highly significant reductions as compared to placebo. The reduction of the risk of progression was 33% and 32%, respectively, for the groups on active drug treatment. Significant reductions in the risk of new brain lesions was also seen in the active treatment groups.

Side effects noted with cladribine included mild to moderate lowering of white blood cell counts, but infections were only slightly more common in the drug-treated groups. Herpes zoster infections occurred in both dosage groups, but were typical "dermatomal" types. Neoplasms were seen only in the drug-treated groups (in 1.4% and 0.9%). There were three cases of cancer in the low-dose group (one case of melanoma, one case of pancreatic cancer, and one case of ovarian cancer), and two cases of cancer in the higher-dose group (one case of early cervical cancer and one case of choriocarcinoma). It is anticipated that approval of cladribine may occur within the next several months in the United States.

Fingolimod has a unique mechanism of action. The drug occupies an important location in the lymphocyte membrane. When phosphorylated, the molecular component representing a lymphocyte receptor effectively submerges into the membrane. This action makes it impossible for activated lymphocytes to exit lymph nodes and participate in immune reactions. In MS, it means that activated lymphocytes that might target the brain or spinal cord are prevented from leaving lymph nodes.

Positive findings related to fingolimod have also emerged from two large trials, including a head-to-head trial with interferon-beta-1a (Avonex). A third U.S. trial should be completed in 2010. In the 1-year international drug comparison trial, annual rates of relapse were 0.33 for Avonex versus 0.15 and 0.20 (significantly reduced) for the low- and high-dose groups of fingolimod, respectively. A higher proportion of patients (83% in the low-dose group and 80% in the high-dose group) were relapse-free on fingolimod versus 69% of patients taking Avonex. However, no difference in disease progression was seen in this short trial.

In both fingolimod trials, transient bradycardia (slowed heart rate) was seen upon administration of the first dose and low-grade (first- and second-degree) heart block was occasionally observed. The rate of herpes infections averaged 5.5% in both trials. Two fatalities occurred from primary infections in the comparison trial, both in the high-dose fingolimod group. One infection involved primary varicella zoster and the other involved herpes simplex encephalitis. Macular edema occurred in four patients in the high-dose group, but was not noted in the lower-dose group.

In the second study, which consisted of a double-blind, placebo-controlled, 2-year trial, highly significant relative risk relapse reductions of 54% and 60% for the two dose groups (high and low, respectively) were found. Significant reductions in sustained 3-month disease progression (17.7% and 16.7%, respectively) for fingolimod versus 24.1% for placebo were also found. The MRI burden of disease was significantly reduced in the fingolimod-treated group but increased in the placebo group. Adverse events were similar in all three groups, but herpes zoster infection occurred in 10 drug recipient patients. Two cases of herpes simplex infection were classified as serious (one labial and one genital), but neither proved fatal. Macular edema occurred

Treatment of Multiple Sclerosis

in seven patients in the high-dose group. In both groups, transient bradycardia (slowed heart rate) was seen in seven patients (two symptomatic) with administration of the first dose. Second-degree heart block was occasionally seen.

It is clear that, as with natalizumab (Tysabri) and other drugs, side effects—sometimes serious—may occur with fingolimod. The similarity of the benefit for relapse reduction with the higher and lower doses of fingolimod, together with the higher incidence of herpetic infections as well as the occurrence of macular edema with the higher dose, will eliminate the higher dose from consideration of approval. The additional safety data from the U.S. fingolimod study (FREEDOMS II) will add substantially to the safety database for fingolimod. With these data, the risk–benefit balance can be ascertained with greater certainty. Approval of fingolimod appears likely, albeit in conjunction with a carefully crafted risk management program.

Additional drugs of MS are currently undergoing trials and should be mentioned. Phase 3 trials of alemtuzimab, a monoclonal antibody directed against the CD52 lymphocyte marker for more active MS (being developed by Genzyme/Bayer), are ongoing. The high incidence of thyroid disease and the occurrence of idiopathic thrombocytopenia (ITP), a serious bleeding disease, complicate this drug's side-effect profile. If approved, its use will likely be limited to major medical centers, which are the only facilities likely to provide the risk management needed.

Rituximab (*Rituxan*) targets lymphocytes bearing the CD20 marker (the earliest marker for cells that eventually produce antibody-making plasma cells). It has demonstrated strong evidence of efficacy in studies of relapsing MS. New studies with a more fully humanized version of the monoclonal antibody are continuing and initiation of Phase 3 studies is anticipated in 2010.

Fumaric acid (BG12, being developed by Biogen-Idec) is currently in ongoing Phase 3 trials. This drug is already approved as a treatment for psoriasis in Europe. In Phase 2 trials, it has provided modestly better outcomes than some of the current standard drugs for MS. Submission of a marketing application for the MS indication is anticipated in approximately 2 years; at that time, fumaric acid will be on a "fast track" for approval in MS.

Laquinimod (TEVA) is in ongoing Phase 3 trials. Submission of a marketing application for this drug in the near future is likely. *Teriflunomide* (Aventis-Sanofi) is also in Phase 3 trials, albeit at an earlier stage than laquinimod. Its developer is not expected to seek marketing approval for this drug in the near future. Other drugs are also in earlier stages of development of MS but will not be discussed here.

Advances in drug therapy of MS and autoimmune disease continue, just as they have continued for other disorders. Although T-cell vaccination for MS appeared to hold some promise, results from this approach have been somewhat disappointing. The dream treatment of eliminating immune reactions aimed at myelin (a theoretical possibility), if given early in the disease, could result in permanent arrest of the clinical activity associated with MS. Trials of altered nervous system proteins (altered peptide ligands) continue, albeit with seemingly less enthusiasm than in the past. The third-generation type of T-cell vaccine also could theoretically induce permanent immune tolerance and could be a "one-shot cure."

Treatment of Multiple Sclerosis

Work employing oral drugs to immobilize adhesion molecules to replace the use of IV medication (Tysabri) appears to have ended. Preliminary efficacy (Phase 2) trials of a product employed by GlaxoSmithKline have ended as well, and other similar products have not been advanced into clinical trials as yet. Because trials have been stopped, these treatments have no chance of becoming a reality in the immediate future. Attempts to block interleukin-12 (IL-12), a hormone essential to the immune cascade, with monoclonal antibodies also have failed to yield more than modest results and have ended. Because of the need to compare the effectiveness of a proposed treatment with the existing MS drugs, rather than to compare a given treatment with placebo, fewer drugs are likely to enter trials for MS in the future. As stated previously, newer approaches to MS management will undoubtedly arise and will enter trials in the future. Only well-designed trials and assessment in large groups of patients will ascertain their value and safety, and only time will tell if they truly represent safer or more effective treatments.

Studies of the roles played by viral genes and their gene products together, and specific immune human responses to them, could point to specific interventions for MS. Perhaps such studies—for example, using available information about molecular mimicry by an EBV protein and myelin—will identify specific events that can be targeted with therapeutic tools. Supplemented by our finite knowledge of altered immune responses in autoimmune disease, designer therapy should be within reach in the very near future.

Karen's comment:

Unpredictable, unknowable, and uncertain are all characteristics of the future for a person with MS. As a person of reason, I think that these characteristics hold true for every-one, MSers and non-MSers alike. As a person of faith, I believe that there is also hope.

100. Where can I get more information about MS?

It is not possible to discuss all of the aspects of MS in one small volume. The appendix to this book identifies a variety of organizations, Web sites, and publications that can be useful to MS patients and their families.

Karen's comment:

In preparing for updating my comments in this edition of Dr. Sheremata's book, I wanted to be current on which issues were on the hearts and minds (and nerves) of MS patients. Below is my abbreviated list of suggested reading. In addition to researching information that is expressly MS oriented, other subject areas can provide fruitful results, including chronic illness; brain function; diet; physical ther-apy; and pharmaceutical companies.

Hard cover books (and their paperback editions) tend to have information that is less likely to contain the most recent medical news due to the timing required for the publication process. However, there are several books that provide unique perspectives on history, politics, and application for the future of MS (such as Curing MS, *by Dr. Howard Weiner), inno-vative and honest approaches to MS (such as* Climbing Higher, *by Montel Williams), and psychological elements and multiple illnesses (such as* Blindsided, *by Richard Cohen).*

Soft cover books are often up-to-date on scientific and medical information as well as having the benefit of vet-ting by the publisher. For those who want more informa-tion on "alternative" therapies," Dr. Sheremata's book can be supplemented with Dr. Allen C. Bowling's Alternative Medicine and Multiple Sclerosis. *A book dealing with emotional aspects of MS is* After the Diagnosis, *by Joann LeMaistre.* Multiple Sclerosis Manifesto *by Julie Stachowiak is a comprehensive and recent book from an MS patient trained in psychology. Books that are not just about MS or spousal issues per se, but about other areas of chronic illness or life changes that have application to MS patients and their families, include* Beyond Chaos, *by Greg Piburn;* Mysterious Stranger Aboard, *by John and Alice Johnson; and* Surviving Your Spouse's Chronic Illness, *by Chris McGonigle.*

Fiction and poetry are helpful for their content, entertainment, escapism and insights into how we and others see MS. There are books written by authors with MS, such as the thrillers by Stephen White, and books by other authors who are aware of MS nuances such as The Breakdown Lane, *by Jacquelyn Mitchard, and* The Sorrow of Archeology, *by Russell Martin.*

Periodicals and pamphlets from the National Multiple Sclerosis Society, the Multiple Sclerosis Association of America, and other nonprofit organizations are published regularly and contain articles on a variety of topics.

NARCOMS (North American Research Committee on Multiple Sclerosis) publishes a quarterly report on MS and collects data from MS patients to facilitate research. This publication is free for patients who participate in the group's registry. The journal has timely scientific information as well as data about clinical trials in process.

The Internet is a way to learn by researching, reading, and interacting with others. Two ways to be notified automatically about MS news are through enrolling in "Google alerts" and MSNews and Views. For information and notification about clinical trials, the National Institutes of Health (NIH) has a comprehensive database.

As to online research and interaction, a word of caution is in order: Be careful. Look at the sources for dates, bias, disclaimers, funding, and common sense. Medical information from the government (including NIH's PubMed) and established medical, academic and MS organizations is usually reliable and up-to-date.

Treatment of Multiple Sclerosis

Organizations

National Multiple Sclerosis Society (NMSS)

NMSS is headquartered in New York, but has local chapters in most communities. It publishes educational pamphlets and sponsors research into MS. Its Web site, http://www.nmss.org, is one of the few truly helpful Web sites available to MS patients and their families as well as to neurologists and other physicians.

Multiple Sclerosis International Federation

Information about MS in English, Spanish, French, Italian, German, and Russian is available from this organization. International Portal provides access to member MS societies around the world. The Multiple Sclerosis International Foundation's Web site (http://www.msif.org) has a link from the NMSS.

Multiple Sclerosis Association of America (MSAA)

Although a smaller organization, MSAA is another important resource. Its contact information is as follows: 706 Haddonfield Road, Cherry Hill, NJ 08002; telephone: (800) Learn-MS; Web site: http://www.msaa.com.

National Organization for Rare Diseases

This organization focuses on important MS-relevant issues. Its Web site is http://www.rarediseases.org/.

Montel Williams Foundation

The Montel Williams Foundation is a newer organization that is getting a lot of attention. It focuses on research into MS. Its contact information is as follows: 331 West 57th Street, PMB #420, New York, NY 10019; telephone: (212) 830-0343; fax: (212) 262-4608; Web site: http://www.montelms.org/.

Multiple Sclerosis Foundation (MSF)

Established in 1986, the MSF is a national, service-based, nonprofit organization. Its mission is to ensure quality of life through support, educational programs, research into the cause and cure, and investigation of medical and complementary treatment options. It offers a resource-rich Web site, found at www.msfocus.org; a toll-free help line staffed by a peer counselor and case worker; and a multimedia library in English and Spanish. Its contact information is as follows: 6350 North Andrews Avenue, Fort Lauderdale, FL 33309-2130; telephone: (888) MSFOCUS (673-6287).

The Pharmaceutical Industry

Members of the pharmaceutical industry sponsor Web sites that can provide helpful guidance, especially for the products they provide. The companies are listed here alphabetically:

Accorda (Ampyra®; dalfampradine): http://www.ampyra.com

Berlex (Betaseron®): http://www.mspathways.com

Biogen-Idec (Avonex®): http://www.avonex.com/msavProject/avonex.portal

Novartis (Extavia®; interferon-beta-1b; fingolimod): http://www.extavia.com

Serono (Rebif®): http://www.mslifelines.com

Teva (Copaxone®): http://www.mswatch.com/Community/

Publications

The Multiple Sclerosis Diet Book, by Roy Laver Swank and Barbara Brewer Dugan (Doubleday Publishers). This book is based on a lifetime of interest, experience, and study. It is a winner. Dr. Swank has spent his life studying MS.

Glossary

A

"ABC": A commonly used unofficial reference to Avonex, Betaseron, and Copaxone, all of which are approved drugs for MS treatment.

Acinetobacter: A bacterium that infects the upper respiratory tract and that has been hypothesized to be a causative factor in MS by some researchers in England.

Acne: A skin condition common in young people that is characterized by increased secretion from oil glands in the skin, accompanied by formation of comedones (blackheads). These glands tend to become infected with organisms living in or on the skin, making the skin raised and red.

Acute disseminated encephalomyelitis: An acute spontaneous, postinfectious, or postvaccinial central nervous system disease. It is characterized by the simultaneous appearance of nervous system symptoms due to inflammation in the white matter of the brain or the spinal cord, resembling an attack of MS. Unlike MS, this condition ordinarily does not relapse in adults but may occasionally do so in children. It can be very serious, but more often it is a relatively mild illness.

Adhesion molecules: Velcro-like proteins on the surface of white blood cells and other cells that allow them to stick to the lining of veins.

Adrenal glands: Glands of internal secretion situated above the kidneys, and hence sometimes referred to as supra-renal glands. The cells of the cortex (on the outside of the gland) secrete cortisone and other steroid hormones that are important in the body's response to stress. Adrenaline and noradrenalin are other hormones secreted by nerve cells in the center (medulla) of the gland.

Adrenaline: The principal hormone secreted by the adrenal medulla. This hormone is made from the amino acid tyrosine and is not a steroid. It makes the heart beat more forcefully and faster and raises the blood pressure.

Adrenaline secretion is also part of the "fight or flight" response to stress.

Adrenocorticotrophic hormone (ACTH): A hormone made in the brain and stored in the pituitary gland at the base of the brain. It is the only FDA-approved treatment for shortening MS attacks. Also called corticotrophin.

Antibody: Proteins made by the immune system that defend the body against infectious agents. At times, antibody may be directed against the body's own tissues, resulting in autoimmune disease. Antibody is produced when B cells are stimulated by antigen.

Anticholinergic: A descriptor for drugs that block the effect of the hormone acetylcholine in the body. These drugs include atropine, scopolamine, and Ditropan. They slow the heart rate down, dry secretions, and reduce the contractions of bowel and bladder. These drugs produce dryness of the mouth and constipation as common side effects.

Antigen: Any substance (bacterium, virus, or single molecule), usually a protein but sometimes a sugar or fat that stimulates an immune reaction in the body. This immune reaction may result in the production of antibody or a cellular immune reaction.

Antigen–antibody complexes: Immune complexes that form when antibody binds to antigen in the blood. The formation of the antigen–antibody complex usually involves another protein called complement. This is a factor in autoimmune disease.

Arthritis: A term commonly used to describe joint disease causing pain. It should actually be reserved for inflammatory disease of joints, such as rheumatoid arthritis.

Artificial insemination: Achieving pregnancy by artificial means. Most commonly, semen from a male donor is injected mechanically into the woman's vagina and/or uterus.

Autoimmunity: The consequence of the arousal of the immune system leading to antibody production or a cellular (lymphocyte) reaction directed against self. The autoimmune response is an immune response generated against tissues in one's own body (antigens). This response may be anti-body mediated, as a result of antigen–antibody complexes; lymphocyte mediated; or mediated both by antibody and by lymphocytes.

Axon: A nerve fiber arising from a neuron (nerve cell). Signals (messages) arising from one neuron are transmitted to another via the axon.

B

Bacteria: Microscopic infectious organisms that cause a variety of diseases in humans and other species.

Biofeedback: A training technique that enables a patient to gain voluntary control over autonomic function.

Brain-derived nerve growth factor (BDNGF): A specific nervous system hormone that can stimulate repair of the nervous system. It was originally found in the brain, but more recently has been found to be produced by cells causing inflammation in the brain.

C

Cataracts: Any opacification (loss of transparency) of the lens of the eye or its capsule. Cataracts are not considered significant if they do not interfere with vision.

Catheterization (of the bladder): Removal of urine from the bladder by means of a urinary catheter (tube).

Cell: The smallest unit of a living animal. Cells are enclosed in a membrane (the cell membrane). They have a nucleus containing chromosomes, mitochondria, and other "machinery."

Central nervous system (CNS): The brain and spinal cord.

Cerebellum: The part of the brain that controls movement, and enables coordinated movement. It is located behind the brain stem and under the cerebral hemispheres; it resembles a pair of tennis balls stuck to the brain stem.

Cerebral cortex (cortex): The layer of neurons covering the entire outside surface of the brain. It appears gray as compared with the white matter inside the brain.

Cerebrospinal fluid (CSF): Fluid produced by the choroid plexus within the brain. It is located in the ventricles and surrounds the brain and spinal cord.

Cervical spondylosis: A disease in which the disks between the vertebral bodies in the neck extrude like mortar between bricks. Sometimes the disks will compress the spinal cord, producing "MS-like" symptoms of weakness and loss of sensation in the legs. The disease process can result in pressure on nerve roots as they leave the spinal canal, resulting in weakness and/or pain in the arms and hands.

Charcot's triad: A collection of symptoms, including nystagmus (shaky eyes), dysarthria, and tremor (slurred speech and shaking of the hands and body) that was described as being characteristic of MS. Although it does occur in MS, it is rare.

Chemotherapy: Treatment with chemicals, such as those that are used for cancer. Examples include cyclophosphamide (Cytoxan) and 6-mercaptopurine.

Chlamydia pneumoniae: A bacterium that can cause pneumonia and that has been studied as a potential factor in MS as well as some other diseases. It is not the organism that causes genital infections in men and women.

Chromosome: Structures located within the nucleus of each cell that hold genetic material. Each human female cell contains 23 pairs of homologous chromosomes: 22 pairs of autosomes and 1 pair of X chromosomes. The human male contains the same 22 pairs of autosomes but only 1 X chromosome that is paired with 1 Y chromosome.

Clinically isolated syndrome (CIS): Optic neuritis, acute vertigo or other isolated brain stem symptoms, or transverse myelitis. These symptoms may be considered diagnostic for MS when certain MRI abnormalities are present.

Clitoral engorgement: Blood flow to the female sexual organ, the clitoris, that is associated with sexual excitement and results in clitoral enlargement (engorgement). It ultimately improves arousal and orgasm (sexual climax) in women.

Cognition: The ability to reason.

Cortisol: The primary steroid hormone (17-hydroxy-corticoid) produced by the adrenal gland. It is the biologically active soluble form of cortisone.

Cortisone: The stored form of cortisol produced by the adrenal cortex.

Crohn's disease: An autoimmune inflammatory disease that principally, but not exclusively, affects the small bowel. It occurs with increased frequency in MS patients.

Cystitis: Inflammation of the bladder associated with symptoms of urinary frequency and urgency.

Cytomegaloviruses: A family of herpesviruses that inhabit the urinary tract of almost all humans. Several subtypes have been described and appear to have geographic distributions.

D

Demyelinating disease: Disease primarily associated with damage to (demyelination of) myelin, such as acute disseminated encephalomyelitis and MS.

Demyelination: The loss of myelin surrounding the axon, or nerve fiber, regardless of the disease process.

Dental amalgam: The material dentists used for dental repairs (dental fillings).

Detrusor muscle: The muscle of the urinary bladder that forms the actual storage organ and is the largest part of the bladder.

Distemper: Illness in dogs and cats caused by the measles-like distemper paramyxovirus of the same name.

Dysarthria: Slurred speech.

Dystonia: Abnormal muscle tone usually resulting in an abnormal position (posture) relative to the rest of the body.

E

Encephalomyelitis: An illness associated with inflammation of the brain and spinal cord.

Enemas: Liquids that are used to facilitate bowel evacuation; usually water- or oil-based materials. They are put into the rectum via an enema tube attached to a bag or other container.

Environmental factor: Any factor in the environment that may contribute to the risk of a disease, such as MS. The environmental factor in MS is assumed to be a virus.

Epilepsy: A brain disorder that occurs when the electrical signals in the brain are disrupted, leading to a seizure. Seizures can cause brief changes in a person's body movements, awareness, emotions, and senses. Some people may have only a single seizure during their lives, which does not mean that a person has epilepsy. People with epilepsy have repeated seizures. Epileptic seizures eventually occur in 1 of 10 patients with MS.

Epstein-Barr virus (EBV): A member of the herpesvirus family that is one of the most common viruses infecting humans. The virus occurs worldwide, and most people become infected with it sometime during their lives. In the United States, as many as 95% of adults between 35 and 40 years of age have been infected with EBV. Infants become susceptible to EBV as soon as maternal antibody protection (present at birth) disappears. Many children become infected with EBV, and these infections usually cause no symptoms or are indistinguishable from the other mild, brief illnesses of childhood. In the United States and other developed countries, many persons are not infected with EBV in their childhood years. When infection with EBV occurs during adolescence or young adulthood, it causes infectious mononucleosis 35 to 50% of the time.

Erectile dysfunction: The repeated inability to get or keep an erection firm enough to complete sexual intercourse. The word "impotence" is used to describe other problems that interfere with sexual intercourse and reproduction, such as lack of sexual desire and problems with ejaculation or orgasm. Using the term "erectile dysfunction" makes it clear that those other problems are not involved.

Estrogen: The steroid produced by the ovary that is responsible for the secondary sexual characteristics of adult females.

Extended Disability Status Scale (EDSS): A grading scale for recording levels of neurologic disability, which was originally developed by Kurtzke. It is used universally for recording disability.

F

Familial infantile spastic paraplegia: A group of different genetic disorders that cause spasticity in family members, usually occurring in infancy. Early onset in a family setting ordinarily easily distinguishes these rare disorders from MS.

Fatigability: The loss of muscle strength following repeated use or testing of one or more muscles. In the clinical neurological examination, the inability to continue walking at least 500 meters is interpreted as a meaningful degree of fatigability of the lower extremities (legs). This factor is used by the U.S. Social Security Administration for disability determinations.

Fatigue: A type of tiredness that is different from drowsiness. Drowsiness is feeling the need to sleep, whereas fatigue is a lack of energy and motivation. Apathy (a feeling of indifference or not caring about what happens) and drowsiness can be symptoms of fatigue. Fatigue can be normal after physical exertion or because of lack of sleep. When persistent fatigue is not relieved by enough sleep, good nutrition, or a low-stress environment, it should be investigated. Because fatigue is a common complaint, associated illness may be overlooked. It is a common symptom in MS and other autoimmune disorders. However, there are many other possible physical and psychological causes of fatigue including anemia, hypothyroidism, infections, sleep disorders, depression, and medications. Chronic fatigue syndrome (CFS) is a condition that starts with flu-like symptoms and lasts for 6 months or more. All other possible causes of fatigue are eliminated before this diagnosis is made.

G

Gadolinium: An injected contrast material used to make blood vessels (or tumors) more visible on MRI brain or other tissue scans.

Gastrocnemius: The large calf muscle that pulls and keeps the foot down (plantar flexes the foot).

Gene: The smallest amount of DNA in chromosomes or mitochondria that codes for a heritable characteristic or feature.

Genetic: Any issue or consideration having to do with heredity, genes, or gene changes (mutations). Also, an inherited characteristic or change.

Genital herpes: A contagious viral infection primarily affecting the genitals of men and women. It is characterized by recurrent clusters of vesicles and lesions in the affected areas and is caused by the herpes simplex-2 virus (HSV-2). Other herpesviruses are responsible for chicken pox, shingles, mononucleosis, and oral herpes (fever blisters or cold sores, HSV-1). Infections with HSV-2 have reached epidemic proportions, with 500,000 people being diagnosed with this

condition each year in the United States. One in five American adults has genital herpes.

Glaucoma: A disease of the eye characterized by increased intraocular pressure causing damage to the retina and impaired vision.

Gray matter: The cortex of the brain; the outermost layer of the brain that is made up of neurons. It completely covers the white matter. The neurons in the cortex send nerve fibers to, and receive them from, other parts of the brain and spinal cord.

Gynecologist: A physician who specializes in diseases that uniquely affect women.

H

Hereditary: Transmitted from parent to child by information contained in the genes. See gene and genetics.

Herpes: Any of several species of herpesviruses (DNA viruses) that are responsible for diseases including chicken pox, shingles, mononucleosis, oral herpes (fever blisters or cold sores, HSV-1), and roseola infantum.

Hormone: The internal secretion of an endocrine organ such as the adrenal glands or ovaries. Hormones are important chemical messengers that communicate with distant organs in the body.

Human immunodeficiency virus (HIV): The virus that causes AIDS.

Hypnotism: The use of suggestion to influence behavior. The field of study that encompasses, among other things, hypnotic trance; its induction, management, and application; and related subjects such as the phenomena of waking suggestion. Hypnotherapy is defined as the use of therapeutic techniques or principles in conjunction with hypnosis.

Hyporeflexic bladder: Decreased bladder reactivity as defined by urodynamic testing in a laboratory.

Hypothyroidism: A disease of the thyroid associated with decreased secretion of thyroid hormone.

I

Immune system: The host defense against infection, which consists of the white blood cells (leukocytes), including lymphocytes and monocytes circulating in the blood and other tissues (including the bone marrow), lymph nodes, and the thymus. Immunology is the study of all aspects of host defense against infection and of adverse consequences of immune responses.

Immunoglobulin: Another word for antibody.

Immunomodulation: Treatment aimed at changing immune responses to benefit a patient with autoimmune disease.

Immunosuppressive therapy: Any treatment that results in decreased immune responses. Commonly used treatments in MS that are immunosuppressive include steroids (prednisone, Medrol, Imuran, Cytoxan, and Novantrone). The interferons (Avonex, Betaseron, Rebif) and Copaxone affect immune responses but are termed "immunomodulatory drugs."

Immunotherapy: Treatment of any kind directed against normal or abnormal immune function, whether involving the products of the immune system or not.

Incontinence: Urinary incontinence; involuntary loss of bladder control.

Infectious mononucleosis: Glandular fever. It is a common form of infection with the Epstein-Barr virus (EBV) and is characterized by fever, fatigue, and enlarged lymph nodes, often accompanied by rash, splenic enlargement, and hepatic enzyme elevation.

Inflammation: The accumulation of fluid, plasma proteins, and white blood cells initiated by physical injury, infection, or local immune response.

Interferons: Cytokines; proteins made by lymphocytes that can induce cells to resist viral replication.

Intrathecal: Inside the central nervous system.

L

Lesion: A localized area of tissue damage, or pathology, of any cause.

Libido: Sexual interest or drive.

Lymph glands: Collections of lymphocytes into organs of immune function; also called lymph nodes. They are numerous in certain parts of the body including the neck, axillae (arm pits), and groin.

Lymphocytes: White blood cells (B cells and T cells); part of the immune system.

M

Macrophages: Monocytes from the bloodstream that have been "turned on" by interacting with lymphocytes.

Magnetic resonance imaging (MRI): Imaging of the brain or other organs obtained by the use of magnetic fields and radio frequency together with computerized tomography.

Malignant multiple sclerosis: A type of MS characterized by frequent, severe relapses with a rapid increase in disability. It constitutes a very small, but important subgroup of MS.

Manic psychosis: A state of elevated mood and psychosis.

Matrix metalloprotease (MMP): Any member of a group of secreted neutral proteases that degrade the collagens of the extracellular matrix. Members of this group are important in the integrity of the blood–brain barrier. MMP9 appears to be the most important of the group in this regard; it is inhibited by interferon-beta (Avonex, Betaseron, and Rebif).

Mitochondria: The cells' power sources. These structures usually are rod shaped but can be round. They have an outer membrane that limits the organelle and an inner membrane thrown into folds from projecting inward (i.e., "cristae mitochondriales").

Molecule: A very small mass of matter; the smallest amount of a substance that can exist alone, which must consist of at least two atoms.

Monocyte: A leukocyte (white blood cell). Monocytes are part of the human body's immune system; they protect the body against infections and move quickly to sites of infection. Monocytes are one of the five major types of white blood cells, and their name is based on their appearance in stained smears under a microscope. They are larger than red blood cells and are typically identified in laboratories (by flow cytometry) by their surface expression of the protein CD14. Monocytes are produced by the bone marrow from stem cell precursors, circulate in the bloodstream for 1 to 3 days, and then typically move into tissues throughout the body. In the tissues monocytes mature into different types of macrophages at different anatomical locations. Monocytes that migrate from the bloodstream to other tissues are called macrophages. These cells are responsible for phagocytosis, or digestion, of foreign substances in the body. An important function is the presentation of partially digested proteins via the MHC class II protein to lymphocytes' T-cell receptors to initiate specific cellular immune responses, as in experimental allergic encephalomyelitis. This effect is thought to be important in MS as well.

Multiple sclerosis (MS): A neurologic disease that is characterized by focal demyelination in the central nervous system and lymphocytic infiltration in the brain, and that has a variably progressive course.

Mutation: A change in the structure of DNA with a potential to alter the normal function of the gene.

Myelin: Lipoproteinaceous material composed of alternating layers of lipid and protein of the myelin sheath.

Myelin basic protein: A structural protein of myelin. It is the most antigenic protein in myelin, meaning it is the most potent protein capable of stimulating the immune system. It is highly effective in minuscule amounts in producing experimental (auto)allergic encephalomyelitis, an experimental form of MS.

Myelin oligodendrocyte glycoprotein (MOG): A specific protein found in oligodendrocytes and in myelin.

Myelogram: X-ray studies of the spinal cord and spinal canal performed by the injection of contrast media. Computerized tomography and magnetic resonance imaging studies have largely replaced this procedure.

Myopia: Short-sightedness.

N

Narcotics: Drugs that produce morphine-like effects. This term is derived from the Greek word for "stupor," and originally referred to a variety of substances that dulled the senses and relieved pain. Narcotics are now defined chemically as substances that bind to opiate receptors (cellular membrane proteins activated by substances such as heroin or morphine). Some people refer to any illicit substance as a "narcotic." In a legal context, "narcotic" refers to opium, opium derivatives, and their semi-synthetic substitutes.

Necrosis: Tissue death; a state of irreversible tissue damage.

Neurologist: A physician specializing in the diagnosis and care of neurological disease.

Neuron: Nerve cell; the morphologic and functional unit of the nervous system. It consists of the nerve cell body, the dendrite, and the axon.

Nucleus: The cellular organelle enclosing the chromosomes. It is bounded by a nuclear membrane.

Nystagmus: Fine rhythmic oscillating movements of the eyeball.

O

Oligoclonal band: Bands of antibody that are present on electrophoresis of cerebrospinal fluid.

Oligodendrocyte: A type of glial cell that gives rise to the myelin sheath. Each cell forms several myelin sheaths.

Ophthalmologist: A physician who specializes in the diagnosis and treatment of diseases of the eye.

Optic nerve: The second cranial nerve, which is actually an extension of the brain. Nerve fibers from the retina travel to the brain through the optic nerve.

Optic neuritis (retrobulbar neuritis): An inflammation of the optic nerve that is characterized by pain and variable loss of vision. Most patients who develop this condition will eventually be diagnosed as having MS.

Orgasm: Sexual climax.

Osteopenia: A lesser degree of bone loss than is present with osteoporosis. Bone densitometry is an accurate way of detecting this bone loss and monitoring treatment.

Osteoporosis: Porous bone; a disease characterized by low bone mass and structural deterioration of bone tissue, leading to bone fragility and an increased risk of fractures of the hip, spine, and wrist. Men as well as women are affected by osteoporosis, a disease that can be prevented and treated.

P

Pathology: The scientific study of disease. Also, detectable damage to tissues.

Pituitary gland: An endocrine gland about the size of a pea that is located at the base of the brain. Its posterior lobe is connected to a part of the brain called the hypothalamus. The anterior pituitary lobe receives releasing hormones from the hypothalamus. The pituitary gland secretes hormones regulating a wide variety of bodily activities, including trophic hormones that stimulate other endocrine glands. ACTH is one of the hormones secreted by the pituitary; it regulates steroid production by the adrenal gland. The pituitary is regulated by releasing hormones from the hypothalamus.

Plaque: The plate-like hardened areas of myelin damage and scarring in MS, which are located in the brain and spinal cord.

Pneumocystis: A one-celled organism that causes rapidly fatal lung infestations in AIDS patients.

Polymorphisms: Referring to genetic polymorphisms, meaning many forms or shapes indicating the presence of mutations, chromosomal breaks, and transpositions.

Postinfectious encephalomyelitis: Acute disseminated encephalomyelitis occurring following an infection.

Progressive multifocal leukoencephalopathy (PML): A serious infection of the brain that is caused by the JC papillomavirus.

Proteolipid: A structural protein of myelin. It can be used to sensitize mice and produce an experimental form of allergic encephalomyelitis.

Pyelonephritis: An acute infection of the kidney associated with fever; it is contrasted with cystitis (a bladder infection), where fever does not occur.

Pyramidal tract: The nerve fiber tract in the brain stem and spinal cord consisting of the nerve fibers that arise from the motor cortex.

R

Rapidly progressive multiple sclerosis: Also known as Marburg's variant of multiple sclerosis; a very aggressive form of MS in which the disease advances quickly and relentlessly, leading to rapid disability and death. It is also known as acute or fulminant MS. Marburg's MS often strikes in younger people and is typically preceded by or associated with fever.

Relapse: Appearance of new signs or recurrence of previous signs of MS.

Rheumatoid arthritis: A common inflammatory joint disease caused by an autoimmune response.

S

Sclerotic: A term referring to hardened tissue, such as MS plaques in the brain. This hardness or sclerosis is caused by scarring.

Seizure: An epileptic event consisting of loss of consciousness usually associated with tonic and/or clonic movements.

Semen: The fluid portion of the ejaculate, consisting of secretions from the seminal vesicles, prostate gland, and several other glands in the male reproductive tract. Semen may also refer to the entire ejaculate, including the sperm.

Shingles: Skin infection caused by the herpes zoster virus. It is typically associated with pain.

Single-nucleotide polymorphism (SNP): Any of a group of gene alterations that may be a "signature group" for a disease.

Spasticity: Velocity-dependent increase in muscle tone.

Sphincter: A circular muscle that constricts a passage, such as the urethra or the anus. When relaxed, a sphincter allows materials to pass through the opening; when contracted, it closes the opening.

Spinal multiple sclerosis: An older term for primary progressive MS, which was commonly used prior to the modern era of imaging.

Steroids: A large family of chemical substances, including many hormones, that are chemically defined as containing a tetracyclic cyclopenta alpha phenanthrene skeleton.

Syphilis: An infection caused by *Treponema pallidum*. Syphilitic infections are similar in type to infections caused by tuberculosis, but are potentially more serious. One type (meningosyphilis, meaning "vascular syphilis") can cause small strokes and its manifestations may resemble MS.

Systemic infection: Any infection that causes generalized symptoms (as opposed to a localized infection). It is usually associated with a fever. Septicemia would be an example of a severe generalized infection. "Sepsis" is a colloquial (slang) term for a systemic bacterial infection of the bloodstream; it is a very serious, frequently fatal condition. Infection with gram-negative bacteria triggers septic shock via tissue necrosis factor alpha (TNF-α or lymphotoxin).

Systemic lupus erythematosus (SLE): A chronic inflammatory autoimmune disorder that may affect many organ systems, including the skin, joints, and internal organs. The disease may be mild or severe and life-threatening. African Americans and Asians are disproportionately affected by SLE. The antinuclear antibody (ANA) test, which helps confirm the diagnosis of SLE, is positive in approximately half of all MS patients.

T

T cell: A type of lymphocyte that develops in the thymus. "Killer T cell" is a term commonly used to describe a cytotoxic T cell. T cells are thymus-dependent lymphocytes that fail to develop in the absence of a functional thymus.

T-cell growth factor beta-1: An interleukin (hormone) produced by lymphocytes that stimulates scarring in tissues. It also stimulates myelin formation.

Testosterone: The principal steroid hormone produced by the male testicles and, to a lesser extent, by the adrenal cortex. It is responsible for stimulating sexual development at male adolescence. It has a positive effect on protein metabolism (an anabolic effect).

Tetanus: A potentially fatal illness produced by infection with the bacterium *Clostridium tetani*, most often complicating wound contamination. It is characterized by rapidly increasing stiffness and may lead to seizures and death.

Thrush: Throat infection by the yeast *Candida albicans*. It is a common complication with treatment consisting of antibiotics and steroids.

Toxoplasmosis: Infestation of the human body by the one-celled organism *Toxoplasma gondii*.

Transverse myelitis: Signs of spinal cord damage appearing acutely or subacutely with signs of inflammation. When accompanied by certain brain MRI abnormalities, it may qualify for a diagnosis of clinically isolated syndrome (CIS) and MS.

Tremor: An oscillating rhythmic movement usually involving an extremity. Head movement may accompany tremor but is termed titubation.

Trigeminal neuralgia: Intense, brief, facial pain typically occurring on one side. It is uncommon before 65 years of age, except in MS. Its occurrence in young adults is usually a sign of MS.

Tuberculosis: The disease that results from infection by *Mycobacterium tuberculosis*. Although this disease most commonly affects the lungs, any tissue in the body can be involved.

Tumor necrosis factor: A principal factor made by macrophages that damage myelin.

U

Urethra: The anatomical tube connecting the bladder with the outside of the body. In the male, it extends to the opening in the penis.

Urology: The field of medical care dealing with diseases of the kidneys, bladder, and associated structures including the ureters and urethra. In men, this field also deals with diseases of the male reproductive organs.

V

Vaccination: The deliberate induction of adaptive immunity to a pathogen by injecting a vaccine, a dead or attenuated (nonpathogenic) form of the pathogen.

Virus: A pathogen composed of a nucleic acid genome enclosed in a protein coat. Viruses can replicate only in living cells.

W

White blood cells: Leukocytes of the blood. A general term used for all white blood cells, including lymphocytes, polymorphonuclear leukocytes, and monocytes.

White matter: A part of the brain largely made of myelin. It gets its name because it contains a lot of fat and looks whitish compared to the cortex.

Y

Yeast vaginitis: A common infection due to the yeast *Candida albicans*.

Glossary

INDEX

A

ABC drugs (Avonex, Betaseron, Copaxone), 11
    for relapsing MS, 125–126
acceptance of diagnosis, 83
accidental trauma, onset or exacerbation from, 74–75
Acinetobacter, 58
acknowledgement of loss, 83–84
acne, 120
ACTH (adrenocorticotropic hormone; Acthar Gel), 11
    attack recovery time and, 23
    for attacks, 115–116
    comparison with steroids, 117–118
    for exacerbations, 100
    function of, 115
    neuroprotective effect of, 113, 114, 116
    recovery time with *vs.* with rest, 118–119
    in reduction and prevention of inflammation and plaques, 11
    for relapses, 113
    side effects of, 119
        comparison with steroids, 122–123
Acthar Gel. *See* ACTH
acute disseminated encephalomyelitis
    CD8+ lymphocytes in, 60–61
    defined, 34
    vs. MS, 34–35
adhesion molecules, 10–11
adrenal glands, 115–116
adrenocorticotropic hormone (ACTH; Acthar Gel). *See* ACTH
advice
    from friends and family, 85
    from medical professionals, 86
AFFIRM safety and efficacy study of natalizumab in relapsing–remitting MS, 127–128
African Americans, 12
age, 11–12

alemtuzimab, clinical trials of, 154
alternative medicine, 148–149
amantadine
    for energy, 91
    for fatigue, 106
antibiotics, for bladder infection, 52
antibody(ies), 61–62
    anti-MOG antibody, 61–62
    defined, 10
    in myelin damage, 8
    NMO-IG, in neuromyelitis optica, 62
anticholinergic drugs, for urinary frequency and urgency, 112–113
artificial insemination, for pregnancy, 94
Asia, 13
asking for help, 81–83
attacks (relapses)
    frequency of, 47, 84
    postpartum, 94–95
    during pregnancy, 94–95
    recovery time for, 23, 113, 118–119
    severity of, 23, 95
    treatments for, 22–23, 95, 113–134
autoallergic reaction, causes of, 60–61
autoimmune disease, connection with virus infection, 63–65
autoimmune reaction, CD4+ lymphocytes in, 60
autoimmunity, defined, 60
Avonex (interferon-beta-1a)
    effect on cognitive impairment, 47
    relapse reduction with, 134
    research on, 84
    side effects of, 125–126
axons (nerve fibers), 4–5
    action of, 4
    defined, 5
    loss of, 5–6
    myelin on, 4, 6–7

B

baclofen (Lioresal)
    intrathecal, for spasticity, 111
    personal experience with, 110
    for spasticity, 108–109

Index